Canine and Feline Respiratory Medicine

Editor

LYNELLE R. JOHNSON

VETERINARY CLINICS OF NORTH AMERICA: SMALL ANIMAL PRACTICE

www.vetsmall.theclinics.com

January 2014 • Volume 44 • Number 1

ELSEVIER

1600 John F. Kennedy Boulevard ● Suite 1800 ● Philadelphia, Pennsylvania, 19103-2899

http://www.vetsmall.theclinics.com

VETERINARY CLINICS OF NORTH AMERICA: SMALL ANIMAL PRACTICE Volume 44, Number 1

January 2014 ISSN 0195-5616, ISBN-13: 978-0-323-26420-4

Editor: John Vassallo; j.vassallo@elsevier.com

Developmental Editor: Susan Showalter

Veterinary Clinics of North America: Small Animal Practice (ISSN 0195-5616) is published bimonthly by Elsevier Inc., 360 Park Avenue South, New York, NY 10010-1710. Months of issue are January, March, May, July, September, and November. Business and Editorial Offices: 1600 John F. Kennedy Blvd., Ste. 1800, Philadelphia, PA 19103-2899. Customer Service Office: 3251 Riverport Lane, Maryland Heights, MO 63043. Periodicals postage paid at New York, NY and additional mailing offices. Subscription prices are $310.00 per year (domestic individuals), $500.00 per year (domestic institutions), $150.00 per year (domestic students/residents), $410.00 per year (Canadian individuals), $621.00 per year (Canadian institutions), $455.00 per year (international individuals), $621.00 per year (international institutions), and $220.00 per year (international and Canadian students/residents). To receive student/resident rate, orders must be accompanied by name of affiliated institution, date of term, and the *signature* of program/residency coordinator on institution letterhead. Orders will be billed at individual rate until proof of status is received. Foreign air speed delivery is included in all *Clinics* subscription prices. All prices are subject to change without notice. **POSTMASTER:** Send address changes to *Veterinary Clinics of North America: Small Animal Practice*, Elsevier Health Sciences Division, Subscription Customer Service, 3251 Riverport Lane, Maryland Heights, MO 63043. Customer Service (orders, claims, online, change of address): Elsevier Periodicals Customer Service, Elsevier Health Sciences Division Subscription Customer Service 3251 Riverport Lane Maryland Heights, MO 63043. Tel: 1-800-654-2452 (U.S. and Canada); 314-447-8871 (outside U.S. and Canada). Fax: 314-447-8029. E-mail: journalscustomerservice-usa@elsevier.com (for print support); journalsonlinesupport-usa@elsevier.com (for online support).

Reprints. For copies of 100 or more of articles in this publication, please contact the Commercial Reprints Department, Elsevier Inc., 360 Park Avenue South, New York, NY 10010-1710. Tel.: 212-633-3874; Fax: 212-633-3820; E-mail: reprints@elsevier.com.

Veterinary Clinics of North America: Small Animal Practice is also published in Japanese by Inter Zoo Publishing Co., Ltd., Aoyama Crystal-Bldg 5F, 3-5-12 Kitaaoyama, Minato-ku, Tokyo 107-0061, Japan.

Veterinary Clinics of North America: Small Animal Practice is covered in *Current Contents/Agriculture, Biology and Environmental Sciences, Science Citation Index, ASCA, MEDLINE/PubMed (Index Medicus), Excerpta Medica, and BIOSIS.*

Printed and bound by CPI Group (UK) Ltd, Croydon, CR0 4YY

Transferred to digital print 2013

Contributors

EDITOR

LYNELLE R. JOHNSON, DVM, MS, PhD
Diplomate, American College of Veterinary Internal Medicine (Small Animal Internal Medicine); Professor, Medicine and Epidemiology, University of California–Davis, Davis, California

AUTHORS

ANUSHA BALAKRISHNAN, BVsc
Resident, Emergency and Critical Care, Department of Clinical Studies-PHL, School of Veterinary Medicine, University of Pennsylvania, Philadelphia, Pennsylvania

VANESSA R. BARRS, BVSc(hons), MVetClinStud, FANZCVSc(Feline Medicine), GradCertEd (Higher Ed)
Faculty of Veterinary Science, Associate Professor in Small Animal Medicine, University Veterinary Teaching Hospital Sydney, The University of Sydney, Sydney, New South Wales, Australia

LEAH A. COHN, DVM, PhD
Diplomate, American College of Veterinary Internal Medicine (Small Animal Internal Medicine); Professor, Department of Veterinary Medicine and Surgery, University of Missouri, Columbia, Missouri

JONATHAN D. DEAR, DVM
Diplomate, American College of Veterinary Internal Medicine (Small Animal Internal Medicine); Staff Internist, William R. Pritchard Veterinary Medical Teaching Hospital, University of California–Davis, Davis, California

STEVEN E. EPSTEIN, DVM
Diplomate, American College of Veterinary Emergency and Critical Care; Assistant Professor of Clinical Small Animal Emergency and Critical Care, Department of Veterinary Surgical and Radiological Sciences, University of California–Davis, Davis, California

HENNA P. HEIKKILÄ-LAURILA, DVM
Resident, European College of Veterinary Internal Medicine (Companion Animals); Finnish Specialist in Small Animal Diseases, Department of Equine and Small Animal Medicine, Faculty of Veterinary Medicine, University of Helsinki, Helsinki, Finland

LESLEY G. KING, MVB
Diplomate, American College of Veterinary Emergency and Critical Care; Diplomate, American College of Veterinary Internal Medicine; Professor, Section of Critical Care, Director of the Intensive Care Unit, Department of Clinical Studies-PHL, School of Veterinary Medicine, University of Pennsylvania, Philadelphia, Pennsylvania

CATRIONA MACPHAIL, DVM, PhD
Diplomate, American College of Veterinary Surgeons; Associate Professor, Small Animal Surgery, Department of Clinical Sciences, Colorado State University, Fort Collins, Colorado

ANN DELLA MAGGIORE, DVM
Diplomate, American College of Veterinary Internal Medicine (Small Animal Internal Medicine); Staff Internist, William R. Pritchard Veterinary Medical Teaching Hospital, University of California–Davis, Davis, California

MINNA M. RAJAMÄKI, DVM, PhD
Adjunct Professor, Discipline of Small Animal Internal Medicine, Department of Equine and Small Animal Medicine, Faculty of Veterinary Medicine, University of Helsinki, Helsinki, Finland

NICKI REED, BVM&S, Cert VR, MRCVS
Diplomate, Royal College of Veterinary Surgeons, Small Animal Medicine (Feline); Diplomate, European College of Veterinary Internal Medicine (Companion Animals); Senior Lecturer in Internal Medicine and Head of the Feline Clinic, The Hospital for Small Animals, Easter Bush Veterinary Centre, The University of Edinburgh, Roslin, Midlothian, Scotland, United Kingdom

CAROL R. REINERO, DVM, PhD
Diplomate, American College of Veterinary Internal Medicine (Small Animal Internal Medicine); Associate Professor and Director, Comparative Internal Medicine Laboratory, Department of Veterinary Medicine and Surgery, College of Veterinary Medicine, University of Missouri, Columbia, Missouri

ELIZABETH ROZANSKI, DVM
Diplomate, American College of Veterinary Emergency and Critical Care; Diplomate, American College of Veterinary Internal Medicine (Small Animal Internal Medicine); Associate Professor, Section of Critical Care, Tufts Cummings School of Veterinary Medicine, North Grafton, Massachusetts

JESSICA J. TALBOT, BSc(vet)(hons)
Faculty of Veterinary Science, University Veterinary Teaching Hospital, The University of Sydney, Sydney, New South Wales, Australia

JULIE E. TRZIL, DVM
Comparative Internal Medicine Laboratory, Resident, Department of Veterinary Medicine and Surgery, College of Veterinary Medicine, University of Missouri, Columbia, Missouri

Contents

the disease. The cause is largely unknown, but it is likely to arise from interplay between genetic and environmental factors. CIPF shares several features with human idiopathic pulmonary fibrosis. This article summarizes the current literature; describes the findings in physical examination, arterial blood gas analysis, bronchoscopy, bronchoalveolar lavage, diagnostic imaging, and histopathology; compares the canine and human diseases; gives an overview of potential treatments; and discusses biomarker research.

Jonathan D. Dear

Bacterial pneumonia is a common clinical diagnosis in dogs but seems to occur less commonly in cats. Underlying causes include viral infection, aspiration injury, and foreign body inhalation. Identification of the organisms involved in disease, appropriate use of antibiotics and adjunct therapy, and control of risk factors for pneumonia improve management.

Steven E. Epstein

Exudative pleural diseases are a common cause of respiratory distress and systemic illness in dogs and cats. This article addresses the pathophysiology, development, and classification of exudative pleural effusions. The most current diagnostic strategies, causes, imaging findings, and medical or surgical treatment options for select diseases are reviewed in detail.

VETERINARY CLINICS OF NORTH AMERICA: SMALL ANIMAL PRACTICE

Preface
Canine and Feline
Respiratory Medicine

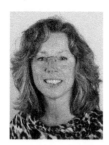

Lynelle R. Johnson, DVM, MS, PhD, DACVIM (SAIM)
Editor

Respiratory medicine remains an underdeveloped field in veterinary medicine. Clinical cases involving the upper and lower airways, lung, and pleural cavity can be challenging to investigate and often require either emergency intervention or long-term management.

This issue of *Veterinary Clinics of North America: Small Animal Practice* brings together a group of talented, practicing veterinarians from academic institutions that has extensive clinical experience in managing cases involving the respiratory tract. Authors share their knowledge with the reader and provide a review of the literature on topics ranging from the newly recognized feline sinonasal aspergillosis to common diseases such as feline asthma, laryngeal paralysis, and canine chronic bronchitis. Each author offers the reader the insight gained from clinical successes and failures in well-written and nicely illustrated articles.

I am ever so grateful to the authors for their devotion to the task set forth and am certain that readers will greatly appreciate the diagnostic and treatment recommendations. Patients and clients will also benefit from the expertise offered by these brilliant clinicians.

Thank you to the production team for creating such a polished final product. Special thanks to John Vassallo, our in-house editor, for his encouragement in completing this issue. Information provided in this volume of VCNA will prove useful for many years to come.

Lynelle R. Johnson, DVM, MS, PhD, DACVIM (SAIM)
Medicine and Epidemiology
University of California–Davis
Davis, CA 95616, USA

E-mail address:
lrjohnson@ucdavis.edu

Vet Clin Small Anim 44 (2014) ix
http://dx.doi.org/10.1016/j.cvsm.2013.09.002   **vetsmall.theclinics.com**

Updates on Pulmonary Function Testing in Small Animals

Anusha Balakrishnan, BVSc[a], Lesley G. King, MVB[b,*]

KEYWORDS

- Pulmonary function testing • Spirometry • Tidal breathing flow-volume loops
- Plethysmography • Arterial blood gas • Capnography • Pulse oximetry

KEY POINTS

- Lung function tests can be divided broadly into those that measure lung mechanics and those that measure gas exchange capabilities.
- Pulmonary function tests do not identify specific diagnoses but instead are used to quantify the severity of respiratory system dysfunction.
- In some cases, these tests are used to determine the anatomic location of disease in the respiratory tract; for example, upper versus lower airway disease.
- The most widely available tool for assessment of pulmonary function is pulse oximetry; however, it provides only a crude assessment of oxygenation.

PULMONARY FUNCTION TESTING

Tests of pulmonary function are widely used in humans in respiratory medicine, sports medicine, and in occupational health. In human and veterinary medicine, pulmonary function testing is used to evaluate patients with known or suspected respiratory disease and is an invaluable tool for assessing the efficacy of therapeutic interventions and determining prognosis. It is also helpful during preanesthetic evaluation of patients and can help identify patients at greater risk for complications.

It is important to remember that pulmonary function tests (PFTs) do not identify specific diagnoses. Instead they are used to quantify the severity of respiratory system dysfunction, and in some cases to determine the anatomic location of the disease in the respiratory tract (eg, upper vs lower airway disease). Widespread use of PFTs is limited by the need for some expertise and specialized equipment to accurately perform and interpret these tests. The application of some PFTs used in humans to veterinary medicine is further hampered because many of these tests require patient

[a] Emergency and Critical Care, Department of Clinical Studies-PHL, School of Veterinary Medicine, University of Pennsylvania, 3900 Delancey Street, Philadelphia, PA 19104, USA;
[b] Section of Critical Care, Department of Clinical Studies-PHL, School of Veterinary Medicine, University of Pennsylvania, 3900 Delancey Street, Philadelphia, PA 19104, USA
* Corresponding author.
E-mail address: kingl@vet.upenn.edu

Vet Clin Small Anim 44 (2014) 1–18
http://dx.doi.org/10.1016/j.cvsm.2013.08.007
0195-5616/14/$ – see front matter © 2014 Elsevier Inc. All rights reserved.
vetsmall.theclinics.com

cooperation and depend heavily on voluntary maneuvers. However, instruments such as blood gas analyzers and pulse oximeters are now readily available in most practices, and this type of PFT can easily be applied to small animal patients.

Tests of pulmonary function can be broadly divided into 2 major categories:

1. Tests of lung mechanics
2. Tests of pulmonary gas exchange

Tests of Lung Mechanics

Lung mechanics reflect the physical properties of the lung and evaluate the relationship between airway pressure, air flow, and lung volumes.

Spirometry

Spirometry is among the oldest and most well-known tests of pulmonary function. The spirometer measures the volume of air or rate of airflow in and out of the respiratory system (ie, volume is measured as a function of time). This method is the accepted standard for diagnosis of obstructive respiratory disease in human medicine,[1–3] and can be used to diagnose airway obstructions in veterinary patients with conditions such as laryngeal paralysis, tracheal collapse, or brachycephalic airway disease. Spirometry can also be used to evaluate ventilatory function in animals with neuromuscular disease, or after anesthesia. **Table 1** lists normal values for dogs and cats.

Spirometry can be performed using a handheld spirometer or a pneumotachograph, which is connected to an endotracheal tube in an anesthetized patient, or attached to a tight face mask fitted over the snout of an awake patient. The pneumotachograph is used to measure flow rates and duration of the various segments of a given breath, including inspiratory time, expiratory time, tidal volume, and peak inspiratory flow (PIF) and peak expiratory flow (PEF) rates.[2] Human patients undergoing spirometry are instructed to take a full inspiration and then exhale forcefully for as long as possible, thereby measuring the forced vital capacity (FVC). Achieving this in veterinary patients is challenging. Therefore, use of spirometry in veterinary medicine is largely confined to tests of spontaneous tidal volumes in anesthetized patients as a measure of neuromuscular function and respiratory drive.

Table 1		
Normal reported values for respiratory parameters in dogs and cats		
Parameter (Unit)	**Dog**	**Cat**
Tidal volume (mL/kg)	10–20	10–20
Minute ventilation (mL/min)	150–250	150–250
Respiratory rate (bpm)	32 ± 10	43 ± 7
Inspiratory time (ms)	920 ± 350	716.6 ± 139.5
Expiratory time (ms)	1170 ± 480	703.7 ± 133.0
Peak inspiratory flow (mL/s)	740 ± 240	110.0 ± 26.6
Peak expiratory flow (mL/s)	780 ± 230	113.7 ± 29.1
Dynamic compliance (mL/cm H_2O)	117 ± 46	19.8
Static compliance (mL/cm H_2O)	42.25 ± 32	NA
Lung resistance (cm H_2O/L/s)	0.8–4.2	28.9

Abbreviations: bpm, beats per minute; NA, not available.
    Data from Rozanski EL, Hoffman AM. Pulmonary function testing in small animals. Clin Tech Small Anim Pract 1999;14(4):237–41.

Tidal breathing flow-volume loops

Flow-volume loops are graphical representations of the relationship between dynamic parameters of airflow and volume during various stages of inspiration and expiration. These loops have wide application and can identify airway obstruction. In humans, flow-volume loops are measured during forced inspiration and expiration. Forced respiratory maneuvers cannot be performed reliably in veterinary patients; therefore, tidal breathing flow-volume loops (as used in human pediatric or neonatal patients) are used instead.[4,5] Airway function in awake animals can be evaluated during tidal breathing by analyzing airflow patterns and waveforms using a face mask. This method is potentially more clinically useful than testing an intubated patient in which the upper airway is bypassed by the endotracheal tube. Causing temporary hyperventilation either by administration of a respiratory stimulant such as doxapram (2.2 mg/kg intravenously) or by temporarily exposing the patient to higher than normal inspired CO_2 levels can help amplify evidence of abnormalities by increasing the changes in air flow and airway resistance during tidal breathing.[6] Induced hyperpnea augments transmural pressure, and therefore exacerbates flow limitation, whether it is intrathoracic or extrathoracic.

To record these loops, patients are typically fitted with a face mask. A pneumotachograph, along with an X-Y recorder to plot a graph, is used to document the relationship between air flow, volume, and time. In awake patients, the inspiratory arm of the loop is negative and the expiratory arm is positive during spontaneous breathing. This pattern is reversed for loops measured during positive-pressure ventilation, when the inspiratory arm becomes positive. Loops are analyzed to evaluate qualitative and quantitative parameters (**Fig. 1**). Qualitative parameters include the overall shape of the loop. Quantitative parameters include:

- Tidal volume (VT)
- Respiratory rate (RR)
- Peak inspiratory and expiratory flow rates (PIF and PEF)
- Midtidal inspiratory and expiratory flow rates (IF_{50}, EF_{50})
- Inspiratory and expiratory flow at end-expiratory volume plus 25% of VT
- Inspiratory and expiratory times

Tidal breathing flow volume loops are useful for detecting changes in airflow in animals with fixed and dynamic upper airway obstructions.[7,8] Fixed upper airway obstructions (extrathoracic and intrathoracic) such as masses cause limitations in airflow (flattening) in both the inspiratory and expiratory portions of the loops. Dynamic airflow obstructions cause more marked changes in one phase of the loop than the other, depending on the location of the obstruction. Dynamic upper airway obstruction such as laryngeal paralysis causes flattening of the inspiratory phase, whereas dynamic lower airway obstruction such as chronic bronchitis causes concavity or flattening of the late expiratory phase of the loop (**Fig. 2**).[7,8]

The usefulness of these loops has been evaluated in healthy cats as well as cats with chronic bronchial disease.[9] Cats with bronchial disease have an increased ratio of expiratory time to inspiratory time, lower expiratory flow rates, decreased area under total and PEF curves, and decreased tidal breathing expiratory volumes (**Fig. 3**).[9–11] This finding has also been shown experimentally in cats that are challenged with aerosolized methacholine, a nonselective muscarinic receptor agonist that causes marked bronchoconstriction.[12]

Lung compliance

Compliance is a measure of the distensibility of elastic lung tissue, and is described as the change in lung volume for a given change in airway pressure. It is typically

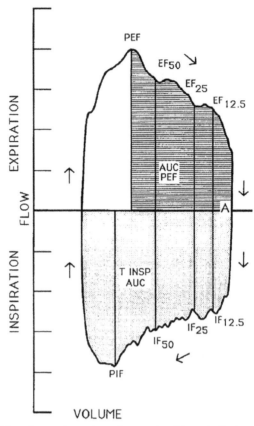

Fig. 1. Tidal breathing flow-volume loop from a healthy cat. Peak expiratory flow (PEF), peak inspiratory flow (PIF), and area under the curve (AUC) are shown. IF_{50}, inspiratory mid-tidal flow rate; EF_{50}, expiratory mid-tidal flow rate. (*From* McKiernan BC, Dye JA, Rozanski EL. Tidal breathing flow-volume loops in healthy and bronchitic cats. J Vet Intern Med 1993;7:390; with permission.)

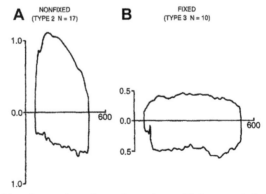

Fig. 2. Tidal breathing flow-volume loops from dogs with laryngeal obstruction. (*A*) A dog with a dynamic laryngeal obstruction. Note the early decrease in peak inspiratory flow. (*B*) A dog with a fixed laryngeal obstruction in which both the inspiratory and expiratory portions of the loops are blunted. (*Data from* Amis TC, Kupershoek C. Tidal breathing flow-volume loop analysis for clinical assessment of airway obstruction in dogs. Am J Vet Res 1986;47:1002–6.)

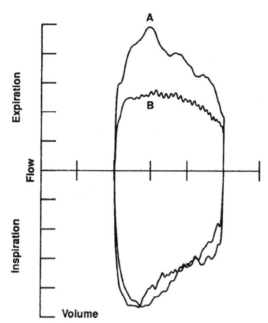

Fig. 3. Tidal breathing flow-volume loops of healthy and bronchitic cats. Note the similar inspiratory flow but marked difference in expiratory flow between normal (A) and bronchitic (B) cats. (*From* McKiernan BC, Dye JA, Rozanski EL. Tidal breathing flow-volume loops in healthy and bronchitic cats. J Vet Intern Med 1993;7:392; with permission.)

expressed as liters per centimeter of H_2O.[13,14] Compliance is routinely monitored during positive-pressure ventilation in veterinary patients. Reported values reflect compliance of both the lungs and the thoracic wall. In order to measure compliance of the lungs independent of the chest wall, esophageal pressure is used as an approximation of intrapleural pressure to calculate transpulmonary pressures. Thus, lung compliance is typically measured in intubated patients. Respiratory volumes are measured by a pneumotachometer that is attached to the endotracheal tube. At points of zero gas flow (ie, at the end of inspiration or exhalation during active breathing, or during a plateau pressure created by an inspiratory hold), pressures measured at the airway are equal to alveolar pressures. Compliance depends strongly on the size of the patient; the lung volume developed by a given airway pressure is much larger in the lungs of a Great Dane compared with a Chihuahua.

Compliance can be either static or dynamic. Static compliance is defined as the change in volume for a given change in transpulmonary pressure, measured when there is zero gas flow.[15] In order to calculate static compliance, airway pressures and volumes are measured during a brief inspiratory hold (plateau). The inspiratory plateau allows redistribution of air throughout small airways that have variable time constants and are slower to open at the end of inspiration.

Static compliance = ΔV/(plateau pressure $-$ PEEP)

where ΔV is change in volume and PEEP is positive end-expiratory pressure.

Dynamic compliance is defined as the change in volume for a given change in transpulmonary pressure during active gas flow, such as during inspiration and expiration in animals on positive-pressure ventilation. Dynamic compliance is therefore the slope of

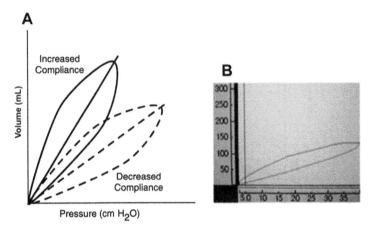

Fig. 4. (*A, B*) Pressure volume loops and dynamic compliance. Note the markedly decreased dynamic compliance (*B*) in a patient on a ventilator. (*From* Corona TM, Aumann M. Ventilator waveform interpretation in mechanically ventilated small animals. J Vet Emerg Crit Care 2011;21(5):508; with permission.)

the line between the two points of zero airflow at the end of exhalation and at the end of inspiration (**Fig. 4**).[15]

Dynamic compliance = $\Delta V/(PIP - PEEP)$

where PIP is peak inspiratory pressure.

In disease conditions in which lung compliance is reduced, higher airway pressures are required to deliver a normal tidal volume. Such diseases include[14]:

- Acute respiratory distress syndrome (ARDS)
- Pneumonia
- Pulmonary fibrosis
- Pulmonary edema (cardiogenic and noncardiogenic)

Lung resistance

Resistance is a measure of the amount of pressure required to deliver a given gas flow, and is expressed as centimeters of H_2O per liter per second.[13] Lung resistance is a function of the nondistensible components of the respiratory system (ie, the airways rather than the lung parenchyma). It is a test of the patency of small bronchi that are deep within the lung. Lung resistance is measured using the same equipment as compliance, namely a pneumotachometer and pressure transducer attached to the end of the endotracheal tube in an intubated patient.

In the normal lung, airway resistance is low, allowing easy flow of air during either spontaneous or positive-pressure breaths. Like compliance, resistance depends on body weight, with higher flow rates expected in bigger animals for a given change in airway pressure. Pathologic conditions that increase airway resistance include those that impede airflow in the small bronchi, such as canine chronic bronchitis and feline lower airway disease (bronchitis or feline asthma).

Whole-body plethysmography

Plethysmography measures total lung volume, functional residual capacity, and residual volume of the lung. In human medicine, it is largely accepted as the gold standard test for determining lung volumes, particularly in cases of airway obstruction.[16–18]

Plethysmography can occasionally overestimate lung volumes in patients that are panting or hyperventilating, with some human studies finding differences of as much as 1 L when lung volumes are measured via plethysmography compared with helium dilution techniques.

Traditional whole-body plethysmography in human medicine involves placing the patient inside a sealed chamber with a single mouthpiece. At the end of normal expiration, the mouthpiece is closed and the patient is then asked to make an inspiratory effort. As the patient inhales against the closed mouthpiece, the chest cavity and lungs expand, decreasing pressure within the lungs. The increase in thoracic volume increases pressure within the closed system of the box, and the volume of the box decreases to accommodate the new volume of the patient's body. The volume within the lungs is then calculated using Boyle's law, which is a useful way of evaluating a patient for objective evidence of lung disease. For example, a large residual volume/total lung capacity ratio with a large total lung capacity indicates hyperinflation, whereas a large ratio with a normal total lung capacity indicates air trapping.[18]

Plethysmography in small animals is challenging because the increase in resistance to flow imposed on the animal during inspiration is usually not tolerated well. Several modifications to this technique have been developed to facilitate its use in small animals.

Barometric whole-body plethysmography In this technique, signals are recorded as a net result of both thoracic and nasal airflow. Exhaled air, which is humidified and warmed, creates a larger pressure change than inspired air even though the flow rates are identical. A pneumotachograph of known resistance is mounted on the wall of the chamber in which the animal is placed, and a pressure transducer is connected to the recording device. The animal moves around the chamber freely and signals produced by inhaled and exhaled air are recorded. The relationship between effort and flow with respect to amplitude and timing can then be evaluated. This technique is useful for evaluating bronchoconstriction in laboratory animals and is well tolerated in small animals, even in cats with asthma that are in respiratory distress.[19–21]

Head-out whole-body plethysmography This modified technique was developed for use in dogs to overcome the tendency of canine patients to pant when in an enclosed box, thereby rendering plethysmographic measurements inaccurate. In this technique, dogs are placed in an airtight glass box that has a fixed volume, with their heads protruding out of the box. A pneumotachograph and face mask are then fitted over the nose and mouth and flow measurements are obtained.[22–24]

TESTS OF PULMONARY GAS EXCHANGE
Arterial Blood Gas Analysis

Arterial blood gas analysis is considered the gold standard test for evaluating oxygenation and ventilation.[25] Samples in small animal patients can be drawn from various locations including the dorsal metatarsal, coccygeal, sublingual, femoral, or aural arteries. In animals requiring repeated sampling, arterial catheters can be placed for easy access. Samples are ideally collected into preheparinized arterial blood gas syringes. All air bubbles should be removed to render the sample anaerobic, and the syringe is capped and processed immediately. Samples can also be collected in regular 1-mL to 2-mL syringes that have been preheparinized by drawing up heparin and then squirting it out immediately. Samples not run within 5 to 10 minutes should be capped to avoid gas diffusion and equilibration with atmospheric oxygen and carbon dioxide (CO_2), and are refrigerated or placed in ice water to prevent cell metabolism, which would distort the results.

A typical arterial blood gas analysis measures the following values (reference ranges for dogs and cats are listed in **Table 2**):

- Pao_2
- $Paco_2$
- pH
- Other acid-base parameters are calculated rather than directly measured, including bicarbonate (HCO_3^-) and base excess (BE)

For proper interpretation of an arterial blood gas analysis, an understanding of the major physiologic causes of hypoxemia is necessary.

Decreased inspired oxygen
Decreased fraction of inspired oxygen (Fio_2) is usually not a clinically relevant cause of hypoxemia unless animals are under general anesthesia and the oxygen valve is accidentally turned off. Decreased barometric pressure at high altitudes leads to lower Pao_2 values in animals with normal lungs because there is less oxygen in inspired air, even though the Fio_2 is normal.

Ventilation-perfusion (VQ) mismatch
This is the most common cause of hypoxemia in animals with respiratory disease. For optimal oxygenation, ventilation and perfusion should be closely matched throughout the lungs. Perfusion of areas of the lung without ventilation, or vice versa, results in inefficient gas exchange, typically hypoxemia. Hypercarbia is less common as a result of VQ mismatch because CO_2 is more diffusible than oxygen. Pulmonary parenchymal disease such as pneumonia or ARDS results in VQ mismatch because alveolar flooding and collapse impair ventilation but perfusion is normal, resulting in decreased ventilation/perfusion ratio in the affected lung regions. In contrast, pulmonary thromboembolism impairs perfusion, whereas ventilation remains normal.

True right-to-left shunting
Anatomic shunts result in mixing of unoxygenated venous blood with oxygenated blood returning to the left side of the heart. Examples include animals with ventricular septal defects or a patent ductus arteriosus that have concurrent increase of pulmonary vascular pressure creating reverse shunting of blood. Intrapulmonary shunting can occur if pulmonary arterial blood is flowing to an area of lung tissue where oxygenation is impossible; for example, a lung mass.

Diffusion impairment
This is caused by abnormalities in the alveolar-capillary barrier resulting in impaired gas diffusion. Diffusion abnormalities are a less common cause of hypoxia, but can be seen in interstitial lung diseases such as pulmonary fibrosis that result in thickening of the alveolar-capillary barrier.

Table 2
Normal arterial blood gas values in dogs and cats

Value	Dog	Cat
pH	7.31–7.46	7.21–7.41
Pao_2 (mm Hg)	92 (80–105)	105 (95–115)
$Paco_2$ (mm Hg)	37 (32–43)	31 (26–36)
Sao_2 (%)	>95	>95

Abbreviation: Sao_2, hemoglobin oxygen saturation.

Hypoventilation
Reduced alveolar ventilation causes hypoxemia, and is seen clinically in animals with upper airway obstruction, respiratory center depression, neuromuscular disease, or severe chest wall or pleural space disease.

Ventilation is a function of the physical ability of the animal to move air into and out of the lungs. CO_2 that is produced in the tissues as a normal by-product of metabolism is eliminated through the airways. Elimination of CO_2 depends on minute ventilation, the volume of air moving through the airways in a given period of time, VT × RR, usually expressed as liters per minute. Because CO_2 is about 20 times more soluble than oxygen, there is a linear relationship between Pa_{CO_2} and minute ventilation. Disease processes that result in abnormal ventilation and can be detected by changes in the Pa_{CO_2} are listed in **Table 3**:

An arterial blood gas sample is the gold standard for assessing ventilation, however if arterial blood cannot be obtained, a venous blood gas can be used. Central venous samples obtained from a large central vein such as the jugular vein or vena cava, or mixed venous samples obtained from a pulmonary arterial catheter, provide the most accurate results. If these are not available, peripheral venous samples can be used to evaluate the pressure of venous CO_2 (Pv_{CO_2}). However, caution is advised in regard to interpretation of these results, because peripheral venous samples reflect CO_2 production in the extremity sampled, rather than the whole body.

Venous samples are not useful for evaluation of the ability of the lungs to oxygenate the blood. Instead, serial measurement of venous oxygen concentrations can be used to assess the ability of tissues to extract oxygen. Poor tissue perfusion can lead to high values for venous oxygen (because it is not being extracted), which then decrease as the tissues become better perfused with treatment. In normal animals, the venous partial pressure of CO_2 is usually about 5 mm Hg higher than the arterial partial pressure of CO_2. This normal arteriovenous gradient occurs because CO_2 is removed from tissues and transported in venous blood back to the lungs as dissolved CO_2 in plasma (about 10%), and buffered within red blood cells as bicarbonate (about 90%). An increased arterial–mixed venous P_{CO_2} gradient can occur in states of compromised perfusion or poor cardiac output.

The approach to assessment of an arterial blood gas sample is given in **Table 4**.

Oxygen Tension-based Indices

Alveolar to arterial oxygen gradient
Oxygenation of blood occurs following diffusion of air across the alveolar-capillary membrane. However, diffusion in normal animals does not occur to a perfect degree

Table 3
Ventilatory abnormalities

Hypoventilation: A Decrease in VT or in RR can Lead to an Increase in Pa_{CO_2}	**Hyperventilation: An Increase in VT or RR Leads to a Decrease in Pa_{CO_2}**
Upper airway obstruction	Pain
Respiratory center depression by anesthetic agents, especially opioids	Anxiety
Respiratory center depression secondary to central nervous system disease	Severe hypoxia
Cervical myelopathy	
Diffuse neuromuscular disease	
Chest wall disease	

Table 4
Steps in the assessment of an arterial blood gas sample

(1) Evaluation of acid-base status

pH		
Acidemic (pH<7.35)	**Normal (pH 7.35–7.45)**	**Alkalemic (pH>7.45)**
Metabolic acidosis?	No acid-base disorder?	Metabolic alkalosis?
Respiratory acidosis?	Mixed acid-base disorder?	Respiratory alkalosis?
Both?	—	Both?

(2) Examination of alveolar ventilation ($Paco_2$)

Increased $Paco_2$ (>45 mm Hg)	**Decreased $Paco_2$ (<35 mm Hg)**
Primary respiratory acidosis caused by hypoventilation	Primary respiratory alkalosis
Compensatory response to a metabolic alkalosis	Compensatory response to a metabolic acidosis

(3) Examination of HCO_3^- and BE

HCO_3^- increased (>24 mmol/L) or BE positive	**HCO_3^- decreased (<18 mmol/L) or BE less than −4**
Primary metabolic alkalosis	Primary metabolic acidosis
Compensatory response to a chronic respiratory acidosis	—

Remember that the body never overcompensates. The primary process can usually be determined by evaluating the direction in which the pH is trending from 7.4. If the pH is less than 7.4, then the acidosis is the primary process. If the pH is greater than 7.4, then the alkalosis is the primary process

(4) Evaluation of oxygenation (Pao_2)

In healthy animals, Pao_2 should be about 4–5 times the Fio_2. When breathing room air ($Fio_2 = 0.21$), Pao_2 should be close to 100 mm Hg. In patients breathing 100% oxygen, Pao_2 should be approximately 500 mm Hg

When Fio_2 changes, equilibration to a new Fio_2 occurs within minutes. Therefore, representative samples can be obtained approximately 5 or more minutes after changing to a new Fio_2

When breathing room air, a Pao_2 of 75–90 mm Hg indicates mild hypoxemia, whereas a Pao_2 less than 60 mm Hg indicates severe hypoxemia because a small amount of blood is shunted to bronchial and pleural vessels, to the coronary venous circulation, and to some areas of dead space ventilation. This normal physiologic difference in the resulting partial pressure of oxygen in the alveoli (P_{AO_2}) and the arterial blood (Pa_{O_2}), namely the alveolar to arterial (A-a) gradient, is about 5 to 7 mm Hg in an animal breathing room air (reference range less than 15 mm Hg).

The P_{AO_2} can be derived from the alveolar gas equation:

$$P_{AO_2} = [(P_B - P_{H_2O})Fio_2] - [Paco_2/RQ]$$

where P_B is barometric pressure (mm Hg), P_{H_2O} is water vapor pressure (mm Hg), and RQ is respiratory quotient (ratio of CO_2 production to O_2 consumption). $Paco_2$ is used as an approximation of alveolar CO_2.

Using an atmospheric pressure of 760 mm Hg, water vapor pressure at 37°C of 47 mm Hg, and a typical RQ for a dog eating normal dog food and breathing room air of 0.9, the equation can be simplified as:

$$P(A\text{-}a)O_2 = 150 - 1.1(Paco_2) - Pao_2$$

The alveolar gas equation and A-a gradient provide a clinically useful method to evaluate the degree of pulmonary parenchymal disease, especially in situations in which the $Paco_2$ is abnormal or variable when serial blood gases are being compared. Because $Paco_2$ is taken into consideration in the equation, hypoventilation or hyperventilation is excluded as a potential cause of hypoxemia. However, VQ mismatch, shunting, and diffusion barriers all cause an increased A-a gradient.

Pao₂/Fio₂

The Pao_2/Fio_2 ratio is another clinically useful indicator of oxygenation status. It is particularly helpful for comparison of Pao_2 values between serial blood gases obtained when a patient is breathing varying concentrations of inspired oxygen. In a normal animal breathing room air with an Fio_2 of 0.21, Pao_2 is between 85 and 100 mm Hg, which results in a Pao_2/Fio_2 ratio of 500.

Abnormalities in the Pao_2/Fio_2 ratio can occur with any type of severe pulmonary dysfunction and are not diagnostic for a specific disease. However, this ratio has been used to characterize the severity of lung disease in animals with acute lung injury and ARDS. In the past, a Pao_2/Fio_2 ratio less than 300 was considered consistent with acute lung injury, whereas a Pao_2/Fio_2 ratio less than 200 indicated ARDS. More recently, the term acute lung injury is no longer recommended and varying degrees of ARDS have been proposed[26]:

- Mild ARDS: Pao_2/Fio_2 ratio 200 to 300 with positive end-expiratory pressure greater than 5 cm H_2O
- Moderate ARDS: Pao_2/Fio_2 ratio 100 to 200 with positive end-expiratory pressure greater than 5 cm H_2O
- Severe ARDS: Pao_2/Fio_2 ratio less than 100 with positive end-expiratory pressure greater than 5 cm H_2O

Pulse Oximetry

Pulse oximetry is a widely available, noninvasive, indirect method for continuously evaluating oxygenation. Ease of use has ensured that this technique has been extensively used in veterinary medicine, particularly in the setting of intensive care units and during anesthesia. Pulse oximetry can be used for measurement of oxygenation at specified time points, as a continuous real-time monitor during stressful procedures, or for immediate assessment of interventions such as oxygen supplementation. If arterial blood samples are not available for blood gas analysis, pulse oximetry can be combined with venous blood gas analysis to provide a reasonable estimate of lung gas exchange function for many animals.

The primary principle behind pulse oximetry is that the concentration of any given solute (hemoglobin, in this case) dissolved in any given solvent (plasma, in this case) is proportional to the amount of light it absorbs. A pulse oximeter probe consists of a light source and a sensor, which is placed over any body part of the correct thickness that has pulsatile arterial blood flow. Common probe placement sites in small animals include the tongue, lips, ear pinna, preputial or vulvar folds, or across digits. Two diodes within the light source emit light of 2 different wavelengths (red, ∼660 nm; and infrared, ∼940 nm) that are specific to preferential light absorption by oxyhemoglobin and reduced hemoglobin. The pulsatile nature of blood flow is detected by the sensor and fluctuations in light absorption cause a rhythmical variation that is then translated into a ratio of oxyhemoglobin to reduced hemoglobin. The hemoglobin saturation of oxygen is calculated from this ratio.[25,27]

A very small amount of oxygen is dissolved in plasma and, in accordance with the Henry law, the relationship is linear. The oxygen content of plasma depends on the Po_2 and the oxygen solubility coefficient (0.0029 mL O_2/dL plasma/mm Hg).[28]

In contrast with the small amount of oxygen dissolved in the plasma, hemoglobin carries most of the oxygen in the blood. The relationship between saturation of hemoglobin with oxygen and Pao_2 is not linear and is shown by the oxyhemoglobin dissociation curve (**Fig. 5**). Each hemoglobin molecule carries 4 oxygen molecules when fully saturated. Binding of the first oxygen molecule causes a change in conformation of the hemoglobin molecule that allows more rapid binding of the other 3 molecules, thereby contributing to the shape of the curve. This curve is shifted to the right or left by several factors such as temperature, pH, and Pco_2, thus altering the ease with which oxygen is loaded onto or unloaded from

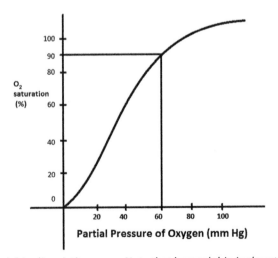

Fig. 5. Oxyhemoglobin dissociation curve. Note that hemoglobin is almost completely saturated with oxygen once the Po_2 is greater than about 70 mm Hg, which creates a safety margin for the patient as hypoxemia develops because of lung disease. However, once the Po_2 decreases to less than 60 mm Hg (which might occur as a result of high oxygen demands associated with stress of handling or transport), severe desaturation is likely.

hemoglobin. The pulse oximeter provides an indirect measure of the saturation of hemoglobin with oxygen.

Although standard pulse oximetry is inexpensive and easy to use and interpret, there are several inherent limitations to the use of this technique. Because only 2 wavelengths are emitted, the device is unable to detect the presence of pathologic variants of hemoglobin dissolved in blood. Any additional hemoglobin species, such as carboxyhemoglobin and methemoglobin, cannot be detected by standard pulse oximeters. This becomes important in the clinical setting in the case of dyshemoglobinemias caused by carbon monoxide toxicity as well as conditions that cause methemoglobinemia, such as acetaminophen toxicity. In recent years, newer pulse oximeters have been developed that emit 4 or more different wavelengths and thus are able to detect additional hemoglobin species that may be present in the blood. These devices are known as pulse CO-oximeters; they measure what is known as fractional saturation, which is oxyHb/(oxyHb + reduced Hb + carboxyHb + metHb), where oxyHb is oxyhemoglobin, Hb is hemoglobin, carboxyHb is carboxyhemoglobin, and metHb is methemogobin.[29] Other factors that decrease the usefulness of pulse oximetry include external motion or noise that causes excessive artifact and signal disruption. Excessive ambient light, especially certain fluorescent lights, can cause erroneous results. Severe anemia can cause erroneously low values, but mild to moderate anemia does not affect the results. Conditions causing decreased perfusion, such as shock or hypothermia, can result in inability to obtain a reading or erroneously low values. In critically ill patients that are anemic, decreased hemoglobin concentration results in markedly decreased total oxygen content of blood. The use of pulse oximetry in these patients can be misleading. Although oxygen saturation might be close to 100%, the total amount of hemoglobin is reduced and the animal can still have extremely low tissue oxygen delivery.[30,31] Pulse oximetry should be interpreted with caution in these animals.

A pulse oximetry reading of 100% correlates with a Pao_2 of about 120 mm Hg,[25] and a pulse oximeter reading more than 95% is considered normal for most animals, correlating with a Pao_2 between 80 and 120 mm Hg. Mild to moderate hypoxemia is indicated by values between 90% and 94%. A pulse oximeter reading of 90% indicates a Pao_2 of about 60 mm Hg. Severe, potentially life-threatening hypoxemia results in Spo_2 readings of less than 90%.

End-tidal Capnography

Measurement of the partial pressure of CO_2 in inhaled and exhaled gases during phasic breathing is known as capnography. This measurement is a noninvasive tool that provides real-time information about ventilatory status, which is particularly valuable for monitoring animals under general anesthesia and for critically ill animals that are intubated and/or being mechanically ventilated.

Commercially available capnometers typically rely on infrared spectroscopy to detect exhaled CO_2 as it flows through a sensor device attached to the endotracheal tube. The amount of CO_2 is estimated by detecting variations in the absorption of light at a specific wavelength (4.26 μm).[32,33] There are 2 main types of capnometers.

Mainstream capnometers

The CO_2 sensor is located directly in the breathing circuit, typically at the hub of the endotracheal tube. Expired air passes directly through the sensor and the CO_2 content is then estimated.

Sidestream capnometers

This device attaches to the end of the endotracheal tube and has a side port through which a small volume of exhaled gas is continuously aspirated. This gas passes through a length of microtubing to a remote sensor in the machine, where the CO_2 content is measured. Sidestream capnographs attached to a nasal catheter have been evaluated in awake, spontaneously breathing dogs, and exhaled CO_2 content correlated well with the $Paco_2$. However, the difference between end-tidal CO_2 ($ETco_2$) and $Paco_2$ is significantly higher in dogs receiving supplemental oxygen, those with tachypnea, or in dogs that have primary respiratory system disorders.[34,35] Thus, documentation of high $ETco_2$ values is a specific indication of hypoventilation, but a falsely normal or low reading might occur in some patients, despite the presence of hypoventilation.

The Capnogram

A typical capnogram consists of 4 distinct phases (**Fig. 6**)[34]:

1. Beginning of exhalation: zero baseline as CO_2-poor atmospheric air from anatomic dead space is eliminated.
2. Exhalation: as CO_2-rich air from the lower airways begins to mix with dead space air, there is a gradual increase in exhaled CO_2.
3. End-exhalation: the amount of CO_2 in exhaled air reaches a plateau during the last part of exhalation as all exhaled air is coming from the alveoli and lower airways. The CO_2 concentration measured at this plateau is reported by the instrument as $ETco_2$.
4. Inhalation: as exhalation ends, the next breath begins and atmospheric air rushes in past the sensor. During this phase, CO_2 levels rapidly decrease and return the baseline to zero.

$ETco_2$ can be used as an estimate of the pulmonary arterial CO_2 because CO_2 is so highly diffusible, and the alveolar CO_2 concentration is normally close to the CO_2 in the pulmonary arterial blood. A gradient between $ETco_2$ and $Paco_2$ occurs because of the presence of dead space:

Anatomic dead space

There is usually a small difference (about 2–5 mm Hg) between $ETco_2$ and $Paco_2$ in normal animals. This difference is a result of some mixing of alveolar air with CO_2-poor air from anatomic dead space in larger airways.

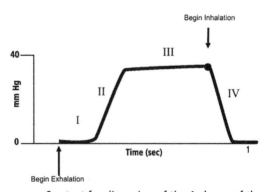

Fig. 6. Normal capnogram. See text for discussion of the 4 phases of the capnogram. (*From* Krauss B, Hess DR. Capnography for procedural sedation and analgesia in the emergency department. Ann Emerg Med 2007;50(2):174; with permission.)

Physiologic dead space

In animals with significant pulmonary disease, the gradient between ET_{CO_2} and Pa_{CO_2} can be increased because of increased physiologic dead space. This increase occurs because some regions of the lungs can have significant ventilation-perfusion mismatch. High V/Q is seen when regions of lung are hypoperfused. As a result,

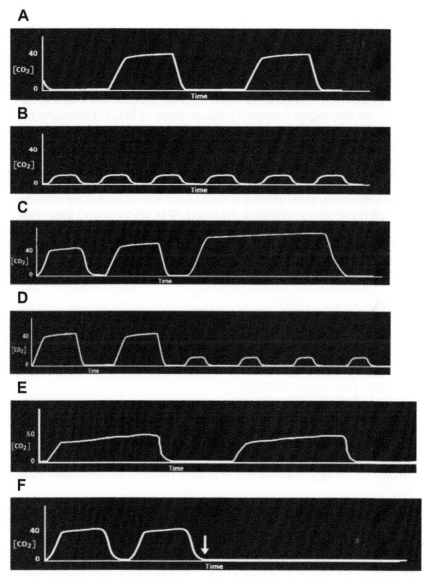

Fig. 7. Capnography during anesthetic monitoring. (A) Normal capnogram. (B) Hyperventilation. (C) Bradypneic hypoventilation. (D) Hypopneic hypoventilation. (E) Bronchospasm (eg, as can occur during an acute aspiration event). (F) Apnea (eg, as can be seen in an intubated patient experiencing a period of respiratory arrest). (From Krauss B, Hess DR. Capnography for procedural sedation and analgesia in the emergency department. Ann Emerg Med 2007;50(2):176; with permission.)

less CO_2 is delivered to that area of the lung for elimination, which translates into a low ET_{CO_2} relative to the Pa_{CO_2}. Low V/Q results when there are regions of alveolar disease. Decreased alveolar ventilation in these areas relative to perfusion results in inefficient elimination of CO_2 and, ultimately, a low ET_{CO_2} relative to the Pa_{CO_2}.

Capnography is an invaluable clinical tool for monitoring ventilatory status. The most common applications of capnography in anesthesia, intensive care, and emergency medicine include:

- Ventilatory monitoring in anesthetized intubated animals[35] (**Fig. 7**)
- Monitoring ventilation in animals with tracheostomies
- Verification of endotracheal intubation during cardiopulmonary resuscitation: attachment of the capnometer to the endotracheal tube after an intubation attempt can help distinguish between accurate endotracheal intubation and a misplaced esophageal intubation because levels of CO_2 in the esophagus are usually negligible, whereas endotracheal intubation should produce a normal capnogram with each breath (either spontaneous or positive-pressure breath)

SUMMARY

PFTs have wide clinical applications and can be used in small animals for evaluation of a wide range of pulmonary conditions. Additional PFTs are commonly used in people but have not found widespread use in veterinary medicine. Impedance oscillometry as a measure of airway function has been widely studied in children with lower airway disease and has potential applications in veterinary medicine because it involves measurements made during normal tidal breathing.

REFERENCES

1. Crapo RO. Pulmonary-function testing. N Engl J Med 1994;331(1):25–30.
2. Morris JF. Spirometry in the evaluation of pulmonary function. West J Med 1976; 125(2):110.
3. Zibrak JD, O'Donnell CR, Marton K. Indications for pulmonary function testing. Ann Intern Med 1990;112(10):763–71.
4. Morris MJ, Lane DJ. Tidal expiratory flow patterns in airflow obstruction. Thorax 1981;36(2):135–42.
5. Carlsen KL, Magnus P, Carlsen KH. Lung function by tidal breathing in awake healthy newborn infants. Eur Respir J 1994;7(9):1660–8.
6. Miller CJ, McKiernan BC, Pace J, et al. The effects of doxapram hydrochloride (Dopram-V) on laryngeal function in healthy dogs. J Vet Intern Med 2002;16: 524–8.
7. Amis TC, Kurpershoek C. Tidal breathing flow-volume loop analysis for clinical assessment of airway obstruction in conscious dogs. Am J Vet Res 1986;47: 1002–6.
8. Amis TC, Smith MM, Gaber CE, et al. Upper airway obstruction: canine laryngeal paralysis. Am J Vet Res 1986;47:1007–10.
9. McKiernan BC, Dye JA, Rozanski EA. Tidal breathing flow-volume loops in healthy and bronchitic cats. J Vet Intern Med 1993;7:388–93.
10. McKiernan BC, Johnson LR. Clinical pulmonary function testing in dogs and cats. Vet Clin North Am Small Anim Pract 1992;22:1087–99.
11. Dye JA, McKiernan BC, Rozanski EA, et al. Bronchopulmonary disease in the cat: historical, physical, radiographic, clinicopathologic, and pulmonary functional

evaluation of 24 affected and 15 healthy cats. J Vet Intern Med 1996;10(6): 385–400.

12. Bark H, Epstein A, Bar-Yishay E, et al. Non-invasive forced expiratory flow—volume curves to measure lung function in cats. Respir Physiol Neurobiol 2007;155:49–54.

13. Rodarte JR, Rehder K. Dynamics of respiration. Comp Physiol 2011;131–44. Available at: http://onlinelibrary.wiley.com/doi/10.1002/cphy.cp030310/abstract.

14. Stahl CA, Moller K, Schumann S, et al. Dynamic versus static respiratory mechanics in acute lung injury and acute respiratory distress syndrome. Crit Care Med 2006;34(8):2090–8.

15. Scanlan CL, Realey A, Earl L, et al, editors. Egan's fundamentals of respiratory care. 8th edition. St Louis (MO): Mosby-Year Book; 2003.

16. Bernstein W. Pulmonary function testing. Curr Opin Anaesthesiol 2012;25:11–6.

17. Rubin BK, Dhand R, Ruppell GL, et al. Respiratory care in review 2010: part 1. Asthma, COPD, pulmonary function testing, ventilator-associated pneumonia. Respir Care 2011;56(4):488–502.

18. Ruppell GL, Enright PL. Pulmonary function testing. Respir Care 2012;57(1): 165–75.

19. Hoffman AM, Dhupa N, Cimetti L. Airway reactivity measured by barometric whole-body plethysmography in healthy cats. Am J Vet Res 1999;60(12): 1487.

20. Hamelmann E, Schwarze J, Takeda K, et al. Noninvasive measurement of airway responsiveness in allergic mice using barometric plethysmography. Am J Respir Crit Care Med 1997;156:766–75.

21. Rozanski EA, Hoffman AM. Pulmonary function testing in small animals. Clin Tech Small Anim Pract 1999;14(4):237–41.

22. Hoffman AM. Airway physiology and clinical function testing. Vet Clin North Am Small Anim Pract 2007;37:829–43.

23. Bedenice D, Rozanski E, Bach J, et al. Canine awake head-out plethysmography (HOP): characterization of external resistive loading and spontaneous laryngeal paralysis. Respir Physiolo Neurobiol 2006;151:61–73.

24. Bedenice D, Bar-Yishay E, Ingenito EP, et al. Evaluation of head-out constant volume body plethysmography for measurement of specific airway resistance in conscious, sedated sheep. Am J Vet Res 2004;65:1259–64.

25. Proulx J. Respiratory monitoring: arterial blood gas analysis, pulse oximetry and end-tidal carbon dioxide analysis. Clin Tech Small Anim Pract 1999;14(4):227–30.

26. Ferguson ND, Fan E, Camporota L, et al. The Berlin definition of ARDS: an expanded rationale, justification and supplementary material. Intensive Care Med 2012;38(10):1573–82.

27. Schnapp LM, Cohen NH. Pulse oximetry–uses and abuses. Chest 1990;98: 1244–50.

28. Habler OP, Messmer KF. The physiology of oxygen transport. Transfus Sci 1997; 18(3):425–36.

29. Yelderman M, New W. Evaluation of pulse oximetry. Anesthesiology 1983;59: 349–52.

30. Hendricks JC, King LG. Practicality, usefulness and limits of pulse oximetry in critical small animal patients. J Vet Emerg Crit Care 1993;3(1):5–12.

31. King GG. Cutting edge technologies in respiratory research: lung function testing. Respirology 2011;16:883–90.

32. Nagler J, Krauss B. Capnography: a valuable tool for airway management. Emerg Med Clin North Am 2008;26:881–97.

33. Sullivan KJ, Kissoon N, Goodwin SR. End-tidal carbon dioxide monitoring in pediatric emergencies. Pediatr Emerg Care 2005;21(5):327–32.
34. Kelmer E, Scanson LC, Reed A, et al. Agreement between values for arterial and end-tidal partial pressure of carbon-dioxide in spontaneously breathing, critically ill dogs. J Am Vet Med Assoc 2009;235:1314–8.
35. Thompson JE, Jaffe MB. Capnographic waveforms in the mechanically ventilated patient. Respir Care 2005;50(1):100–8.

Laryngeal Disease in Dogs and Cats

Catriona MacPhail, DVM, PhD

KEYWORDS

- Upper airway obstruction • Laryngeal paralysis • Aspiration pneumonia
- Megaesophagus • Laryngeal collapse • Tracheostomy

KEY POINTS

- The most common disease process involving the larynx is laryngeal paralysis, which occurs much more frequently in dogs than in cats.
- Diagnosis of laryngeal paralysis requires close attention to anesthetic plane and coordination of respiratory effort with laryngeal motion.
- Surgical arytenoid lateralization improves respiration and quality of life in dogs with laryngeal paralysis; however, aspiration pneumonia is a recognized complication, and generalized neuropathy can progress.
- Laryngeal collapse can result from any cause of chronic upper airway obstruction, but is most often associated with unaddressed brachycephalic airway syndrome.
- Laryngeal neoplasia, while generally uncommon, occurs more frequently in cats than in dogs. Histologic confirmation is required to exclude inflammatory laryngeal disease.

INTRODUCTION

Laryngeal disease in dogs and cats results in varying degrees of upper airway obstruction and can be life-threatening. Conditions most commonly affecting the larynx include laryngeal paralysis, laryngeal collapse, and laryngeal masses. Differentials for laryngeal disease include nasal, nasopharyngeal, and tracheal conditions that also result in clinical signs of upper airway obstruction, such as stertor, stridor, wheezing, and gagging. Visual upper airway examination is the fundamental diagnostic tool for localizing the anatomic area involved in airway obstruction.

ANATOMY AND PHYSIOLOGY

The larynx is the collection of cartilages surrounding the rima glottidis. It is responsible for control of airflow during respiration. The four cartilages that constitute the larynx are the paired arytenoids and the unpaired epiglottis, cricoid, and thyroid

Department of Clinical Sciences, Colorado State University, Fort Collins, CO 80523, USA
E-mail address: Catriona.MacPhail@colostate.edu

Vet Clin Small Anim 44 (2014) 19–31
http://dx.doi.org/10.1016/j.cvsm.2013.09.001   vetsmall.theclinics.com

cartilages. Each of the arytenoid cartilages has a cuneiform process rostrally, a corniculate process dorsally, a muscular process dorsolaterally, and a vocal process ventrally. The vocal processes are the attachment points for the vocal folds. The glottis consists of the vocal folds, the vocal process of the arytenoid cartilages, and the rima glottides. The laryngeal saccules are mucosal diverticula that sit rostral and lateral to the vocal folds. The larynx of the cat differs from that of the dog as the arytenoid cartilage lacks cuneiform and corniculate processes. Also, true aryepiglottic folds are absent and the sides of the epiglottis connect directly to the cricoid lamina by laryngeal mucosa.

The intrinsic muscles of the larynx (cricoarytenoideus dorsalis, cricoarytenoideus lateralis, thyroarytenoideus, vocalis, ventricularis, arytenoideus transversus, hyoepiglotticus, and cricothyroideus) are responsible for all laryngeal functions. These functions include regulation of airflow, protection of the lower airway from aspiration during swallowing, and control of phonation. The cricoarytenoideus dorsalis muscle is solely responsible for enlarging the glottis during inspiration. This muscle originates on the dorsolateral surface of the cricoid and inserts on the muscular process of the arytenoid cartilages. Contraction of this muscle results in external rotation and abduction of the arytenoid cartilages that then pulls the vocal processes laterally. The caudal laryngeal nerve is the terminal segment of the recurrent laryngeal nerve and is responsible for innervation of all intrinsic laryngeal muscles, except the cricothyroid muscle, which is innervated by the cranial laryngeal nerve.

CANINE LARYNGEAL PARALYSIS
Cause

Laryngeal paralysis is a common unilateral or bilateral respiratory disorder that primarily affects older (>9 years) large- and giant-breed dogs. A congenital form occurs in certain breeds such as Bouvier des Flandres, Siberian huskies, bull terriers, and white-coated German shepherd dogs.[1,2] An autosomal-dominant trait has been documented in Bouvier des Flandres, resulting in Wallerian degeneration of the recurrent laryngeal nerves and abnormalities of the nucleus ambiguus.[3] Although the precise mode of inheritance has not been established, a hereditary predisposition has also been identified in Siberian husky dogs, Alaskan malamutes, and crosses of those 2 breeds.[4,5] A laryngeal paralysis-polyneuropathy complex has been described in Dalmatians, Rottweilers, Leonberger dogs, and Pyrean mountain dogs.[6–9]

For the more frequently encountered acquired laryngeal paralysis, the Labrador retriever is the most common breed reported, but golden retrievers, Saint Bernards, Newfoundlands, and Irish setters are also overrepresented. Proposed causes of laryngeal paralysis include accidental trauma, iatrogenic trauma, cervical masses, and neuromuscular disease (**Box 1**). In most dogs the cause remains undetermined, and these cases are traditionally classified as idiopathic.

Recently it was shown that many dogs develop systemic neurologic signs within 1 year following diagnosis of laryngeal paralysis, which is consistent with progressive generalized neuropathy.[10] Abnormalities in the results of electrodiagnostic tests and histopathologic analysis of nerve and muscle biopsy specimens reflecting generalized polyneuropathy have also been documented in dogs with acquired laryngeal paralysis.[11] It has been suggested that dogs previously thought to have idiopathic laryngeal paralysis could in fact have a progressive generalized polyneuropathy. The abbreviation GOLPP (geriatric onset laryngeal paralysis polyneuropathy) has been proposed as a more accurate term for dogs with acquired laryngeal paralysis where other causes have been ruled out.[10]

Box 1
Causes of laryngeal paralysis
Congenital
Accidental trauma
Cervical penetrating wounds
Strangulating trauma
Iatrogenic surgical trauma
Ventral slot
Thyroidectomy/parathyroidectomy
Tracheal surgery
Cranial thoracic surgery
Cervical/intrathoracic masses
Thyroid carcinoma
Thymoma
Lymphoma
Abscess
Granuloma
Neuromuscular disease
Immune-mediated
Infectious
Toxins (lead; organophosphates)
Endocrinopathy
Polymyopathy
Progressive idiopathic polyneuropathy

Clinical Signs

With laryngeal paralysis, the arytenoid cartilages, and consequently the vocal folds, remain in a paramedian position during inspiration creating upper airway obstruction. Dogs typically present with noisy inspiratory respiration and exercise intolerance. Early clinical signs include voice change and mild coughing and gagging. Severe airway obstruction results in respiratory distress, cyanosis, and collapse. Dogs can also exhibit dysphagia or develop rear limb weakness associated with peripheral neuropathy. The classic finding on physical examination is the presence of stridor over the upper airway but this can be variable. A complete neurologic examination and assessment of proprioceptive placing should be performed in dogs suspected of laryngeal paralysis.

Progression of clinical signs is highly variable, and dogs can have clinical signs for several months to years before significant respiratory distress ensues. However, clinical signs are worsened by heavy exercise or increasing environmental temperature or humidity, which results in an acute exacerbation of a chronic condition. As respiratory rate increases, the mucosa covering the arytenoids becomes inflamed and edematous, which leads to further airway obstruction. A vicious cycle ensues that if unaddressed can become life threatening.

Diagnosis

Routine diagnostic evaluation for dogs thought to have laryngeal paralysis includes physical examination, neurologic examination, complete blood count, biochemical profile, urinalysis, thyroid function screening, thoracic radiographs, and laryngeal examination. Dogs with laryngeal paralysis are at risk of aspiration pneumonia both before and after surgery. Therefore thoracic radiographs are a necessary part of the diagnostic workup in dogs suspected of laryngeal dysfunction to rule out aspiration pneumonia, as well as overt megaesophagus, pulmonary edema, and concurrent cardiac or lower airway abnormalities (**Fig. 1**).

For dogs that present with dysphagia or vomiting, an esophagram should be obtained to investigate esophageal dysfunction or megaesophagus, which might not be apparent on plain thoracic radiographs. Severe progressive esophageal dysfunction has been reported in a set of dogs with idiopathic laryngeal paralysis and likely reflects the progressive polyneuropathy that has been proposed as a cause of laryngeal dysfunction in most geriatric dogs.[10]

Hypothyroidism occurs concurrently in approximately 30% of dogs with acquired laryngeal paralysis, although a direct causal link has not been established.[12,13] Regardless, thyroid function screening is performed routinely in the workup for laryngeal paralysis. Thyroid supplementation should be instituted if indicated, although this does not resolve clinical signs associated with laryngeal paralysis.

Definitive diagnosis of laryngeal paralysis requires laryngeal examination. This examination can be accomplished by direct visualization of the larynx with a simple laryngoscope, oral video-endoscopic laryngoscopy, transnasal laryngoscopy, ultrasound (echolaryngography), or computed tomography (CT). Findings indicate laryngeal paralysis on ultrasound, including asymmetry or absence of motion of the cuneiform processes, abnormal arytenoid movement, paradoxic movement, caudal displacement of the larynx, and laryngeal collapse.[14] CT findings in dogs with laryngeal paralysis included failure to abduct the arytenoid cartilages and collapse into the rima glottis on presumed inspiration, stenosis of the laryngeal inlet, and air-filled lateral ventricles.[15] Laryngoscopy, regardless of method, can be confounding as false-positive results are common due to the influence of anesthetic agents and sedatives on laryngeal function. Echolaryngography, transnasal laryngoscopy, and CT avoid the need for heavy sedation and general anesthesia; however, none of these methods have been shown to be superior to traditional oral laryngeal examination for definitive diagnosis.[16]

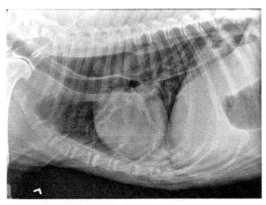

Fig. 1. Lateral thoracic radiograph of a dog with laryngeal paralysis showing megaesophagus.

Laryngeal paralysis is diagnosed based on the lack of arytenoid abduction during inspiration. Inflammation and swelling of the laryngeal cartilages can also be apparent. Diagnosis can be confounded by paradoxic movement of the arytenoids, resulting in a false-negative result. In this scenario, the arytenoid cartilages move inward during inspiration because of negative intraglottic pressure created by breathing against an obstruction. The cartilages then passively return to a normal position during expiration, which gives the impression of normal arytenoid movement. To avoid this situation, an assistant should state the phase of ventilation during laryngoscopy to help in distinguishing normal from abnormal motion.

Intravenous thiopental administered to effect is thought to be the best anesthetic choice for assessment of laryngeal function.[17] However, the recent lack of availability of thiopental leaves propofol as the most appropriate induction agent for laryngeal examination in dogs (**Box 2**). Doxapram HCl (1 mg/kg IV) has been advocated for routine use during laryngoscopy to increase respiratory rate and effort and improve intrinsic laryngeal motion, and it should be administered if the diagnosis is in doubt.[18,19]

Emergency Treatment

For dogs in acute respiratory distress associated with airway obstruction, initial treatment is directed at improving ventilation, reducing laryngeal edema, and minimizing the animal's stress. A typical treatment regimen involves oxygen supplementation and administration of short-acting steroids (eg, dexamethasone 0.1–1 mg/kg IV) and sedatives (eg, acepromazine 0.02 mg/kg IV). Additional administration of buprenorphine (0.005 mg/kg IV) or butorphanol (0.2 mg/kg IV) can also be considered to improve sedation. These dogs are often hyperthermic because of excessive respiratory effort, and appropriate cooling procedures should also be instituted including wetting the fur with cool water and application of a fan. If respiratory distress cannot be abated, intubation or a temporary tracheostomy should be considered. However, use of a temporary tracheostomy tube in dogs with laryngeal paralysis has been shown to be a negative prognostic indicator following surgery, because dogs that received a temporary tracheostomy preoperatively were more likely to experience major complications.[13]

Box 2
Drugs used during functional laryngeal examination

Premedications:

Glycopyrrolate: 0.005–0.01 mg/kg IV, IM, SC *and*

Butorphanol: 0.2–0.4 mg/kg IV, IM, SQ *or*

Buprenorphine: 0.005–0.02 mg/kg IV, IM, SC *or*

Hydromorphone: 0.1–0.2 mg/kg IV, IM, SC

Induction:

Propofol: 4–8 mg/kg IV, administered slowly

To stimulate respiration:

Doxapram HCl: 1–2 mg/kg IV

To decrease laryngeal swelling:

Dexamethasone: 0.1–1 mg/kg IV

Temporary tracheostomies are not without complications. The presence of a tube within the tracheal lumen causes epithelial erosion, submucosal inflammation, and inhibition of the mucociliary apparatus. Mucus production dramatically increases, and the tube must be suctioned or cleaned at very frequent intervals to prevent clogging. Therefore, a dog with a temporary tracheostomy tube requires intensive monitoring to avoid life-threatening complications. In a recent study, complications (clinical and incidental) were documented in 86% of cases receiving a temporary tracheostomy.[20] Sixteen types of complications were noted, but the most significant and frequent complications occurred in ~25% of dogs and were airway obstruction, tube dislodgement, aspiration pneumonia, and stoma swelling.

Medical Management

Often dogs are not severely affected clinically until they have bilateral laryngeal paresis or paralysis. Therefore, dogs with unilateral laryngeal dysfunction are typically not surgical candidates. For dogs with bilateral laryngeal paralysis, the decision to recommend surgery is based on the quality of life of the dog, severity of clinical signs, and time of year. The goal of conservative management of dogs with laryngeal paralysis is to improve the quality of life through environmental changes, reduction of daily exercise, owner education, weight loss, and consideration of anti-inflammatory drugs to minimize laryngeal swelling. Unfortunately, medical treatment is insufficient for long-term management. For dogs that are diagnosed with concurrent hypothyroidism, thyroid supplementation should be instituted, but as noted earlier this rarely improves clinical signs of laryngeal paralysis but can assist with weight loss.

Surgical Treatment

Laryngeal paralysis is a surgical condition for severely affected dogs, and numerous techniques have been described. Unilateral arytenoid lateralization is the current technique of choice for most surgeons but various types of partial laryngectomy (bilateral vocal fold resection, partial arytenoidectomy) are also performed. Bilateral arytenoid lateralization is not recommended because it results in unacceptable morbidity.[13] Other techniques include castellated laryngofissure, reinnervation of the laryngeal musculature, and permanent tracheostomy. Castellated laryngofissure is performed rarely because of the technical difficulty of the procedure and inconsistent outcomes. Reinnervation does not provide immediate clinical relief, so it is not a practical treatment option in dogs. Permanent tracheostomy is considered a salvage procedure for dogs most at risk of aspiration pneumonia, but it is associated with a high rate of major and minor complications and requires diligent postoperative and long-term care. Also, the risk for aspiration pneumonia remains despite the presence of a permanent stoma.

Several variations of unilateral arytenoid lateralization have been described. The most common technique involves suturing the cricoid cartilage to the muscular process of the arytenoid cartilage. This technique mimics the directional pull of the cricoarytenoideus dorsalis muscle and rotates the arytenoid cartilage laterally. An alternative technique involves suture placement from the muscular process of the arytenoid cartilage to the caudodorsal aspect of the thyroid cartilage. This technique pulls the arytenoid cartilage laterally rather than rotating it and increases the area of the rima glottidis to a lesser degree than the cricoarytenoid suture. Differences in surgical technique and the degree of increase in surface area of the rima glottis do not seem to affect postoperative clinical signs and outcome. However, increasing the surface area of the rima glottidis beyond the edges of the epiglottis could put the animal at higher risk of aspiration. Limited lateral displacement of the arytenoid cartilage will significantly reduce airway resistance within the larynx and might decrease the risk of postoperative aspiration pneumonia.[21] This lateral displacement can be accomplished by minimizing the degree of dissection: separation of the cricothyroid articulation, transection of the sesamoid band connecting the paired arytenoids, and complete disarticulation of the cricoarytenoid joint are not necessary. A partial opening of the cricoarytenoid articulation allows accurate visualization of needle placement through the muscular process of the arytenoid but limits the degree of arytenoid cartilage abduction.

Partial laryngectomy encompasses various techniques for vocal cord excision and partial arytenoidectomy to increase the diameter of the glottis. Partial laryngectomy has been associated with complications, including laryngeal webbing, laryngeal scarring, and aspiration pneumonia. High complication rates have been reported; however, bilateral vocal fold resection alone resulted in fewer complications and better postoperative outcome than other partial laryngectomy techniques.[13,22–24] Bilateral vocal fold excision and thyroarytenoid lateralization performed through a ventral laryngotomy improves clinical signs and is associated with a low rate of aspiration pneumonia; however, recurrence of clinical signs is common, likely because of narrowing of the rima glottis.[25] Successful partial arytenoidectomy by photoablation of the left arytenoid cartilage tissue using a diode laser has been reported in a small set of dogs.[26] Recently, bilateral ventriculocordectomy via ventral laryngotomy was reported to have a reasonable long-term (>6 months) outcome with a low incidence of major complication (7%).[24]

Prognosis

Aspiration pneumonia is the most common complication in dogs surgically treated for laryngeal paralysis; it occurs in 10% to 21% of dogs undergoing unilateral arytenoid lateralization.[13,27,28] Although aspiration pneumonia is most likely in the first few weeks following surgery, dogs are at risk of this complication for the rest of their lives.[13] Factors that have been found to be significantly associated with a higher risk of developing complications and a negative effect on long-term outcome include preoperative aspiration pneumonia, development of esophageal dysfunction, progression of generalized neurologic signs, temporary tracheostomy placement, and concurrent neoplastic disease.[13] In one study, 10 of 32 dogs had neurologic signs at the time of enrollment into the study, but all dogs had neurologic signs by 1 year.[10]

In the absence of surgical complications, unilateral arytenoid lateralization results in less respiratory distress, less respiratory noise, and improved exercise tolerance. Owner satisfaction with this procedure has been reported as excellent, with most owners believing that the quality of the dog's life was improved dramatically.[13,27]

FELINE LARYNGEAL PARALYSIS

Laryngeal disease is uncommon in cats, but significant respiratory stress can result. In a review of laryngeal diseases in cats, laryngeal paralysis constituted 40% of cases.[29] Clinical presentation is similar to dogs in that it occurs most often in middle-aged to older cats (mean 9–14 years) and both unilateral and bilateral conditions have been documented. Significant unilateral dysfunction has been reported in 10% to 57% of cases.[29–31] There is also a predominance of left-sided unilateral laryngeal paralysis in cats, which is similar to that reported in humans and horses. Clinical signs and physical examination findings resemble those found in dogs, with inspiratory respiratory difficulty, change in meow, gagging, and stridor found most commonly.

The specific cause of laryngeal paralysis in cats often remains undetermined. Several cases have been reported in association with trauma, neoplastic invasion, and iatrogenic damage to the recurrent laryngeal nerve (eg, postthyroidectomy). Neoplastic infiltration of the larynx can lead to fixed laryngeal obstruction with both inspiratory and expiratory dyspnea and noise and should always be considered in the differential diagnosis of laryngeal paralysis in the cat. In addition to traditional laryngoscopy (direct or endoscopically), the use of echolaryngography has been described for diagnosis of laryngeal paralysis in cats.[29,32]

Conservative management of cats with laryngeal paralysis consists of weight loss and minimization of excitement and rigorous exercise. Reported survival times in 7 cats treated conservatively for laryngeal paralysis ranged from 120 to 2520 days with a median survival of 811 days.[29] Successful surgical treatment using primarily unilateral arytenoid lateralization has been described in several small studies with reported median survival time of approximately 150 days.[29–31]

LARYNGEAL COLLAPSE

Laryngeal collapse is a consequence of chronic upper airway obstruction, most often associated with brachycephalic airway syndrome. Brachycephalic airway syndrome refers to the condition of obstructive airway distress attributable to anatomic abnormalities of breeds such as English and French bulldogs, pugs, Boston terriers, and Cavalier King Charles spaniels. Chronic upper airway obstruction from the main components of brachycephalic airway syndrome (stenotic nares, elongated soft palate) causes increased airway resistance and increased negative intraglottic luminal pressure. Over time this results in laryngeal collapse because of cartilage fatigue and degeneration. However, early onset of laryngeal collapse has also been reported, with affected brachycephalic dogs ranging in age from 4.5 to 6 months.[33] Finally, laryngeal collapse can also be associated with laryngeal paralysis, nasal and nasopharyngeal obstruction, or trauma.

There are 3 stages of severity to laryngeal collapse. Stage 1 is the eversion of the laryngeal saccules into the glottis (**Fig. 2**). Increased inspiratory effort creates a vacuum causing the mucosa of the laryngeal saccules to prolapse. In most studies regarding brachycephalic airway syndrome, everted laryngeal saccules are present in 50% to 60% of affected dogs.[34–36] The saccules are pulled from their crypts

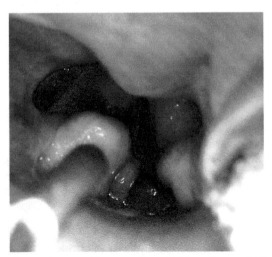

Fig. 2. Severely swollen and everted laryngeal saccules in a 6-year-old English bulldog.

because of the high negative pressure within the glottis. Once the saccules are everted, the tissue is exposed to highly turbulent airflow, resulting in edema and inflammation, which further obstructs the airway. During stage 2, the cuneiform processes of the arytenoid cartilages lose rigidity and collapse into the laryngeal lumen (**Fig. 3**). In addition, the aryepiglottic folds collapse ventromedially. The most advanced phase of laryngeal collapse is stage 3, in which the corniculate process of each arytenoid cartilage fatigues and then collapses toward midline, resulting in complete laryngeal collapse.

Diagnosis of laryngeal collapse requires oral laryngeal examination under heavy sedation or a light plane of general anesthesia without intubation. Functional, as well as structural, examination of the larynx should be performed. Recently, CT imaging with 3-dimensional internal rendering was used in 9 dogs with laryngeal collapse that had imaging performed in the absence of sedation or general anesthesia.[15] Findings consistent with laryngeal collapse included everted laryngeal saccules, collapse of the cuneiform processes and corniculate processes, and narrowed rima glottis.

The early stage of laryngeal collapse is still amenable to surgical treatment. Resection of the everted laryngeal saccules is relatively simple because each saccule is grasped with Allis tissue forceps and then sharply transected with Metzenbaum scissors. Options for treatment of advanced stages of laryngeal collapse are limited. Underlying components of brachycephalic airway syndrome should be addressed and degree of improvement should be assessed. Dogs with stage 2 and 3 laryngeal collapse have been shown to benefit markedly from removal of everted laryngeal saccules in addition to surgical correction of elongated soft palate and stenotic nares.[36] Unilateral arytenoid lateralization has recently been reported to have reasonable long-term outcome in dogs with laryngeal collapse, but this technique should be used with caution as the opposite cartilage can continue to collapse medially, leading to airway obstruction.[37] Permanent tracheostomy is the recommended treatment when dogs do not respond to other medical or surgical treatment, although many owners consider this an unacceptable option because of the high risk of complications and degree of maintenance required (**Fig. 4**).

LARYNGEAL MASSES
Neoplasia

Tumors of the larynx are uncommon in the dog and cat. Numerous types of tumor have been reported in the dog, including rhabdomyosarcoma (oncocytoma), squamous cell

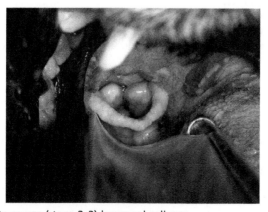

Fig. 3. Moderate to severe (stage 2–3) laryngeal collapse.

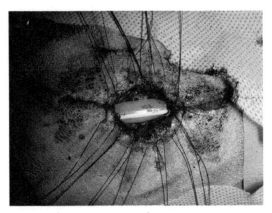

Fig. 4. Intraoperative view of a permanent tracheostomy.

carcinoma, adenocarcinoma, osteosarcoma, chondrosarcoma, fibrosarcoma, plasmacytoma, undifferentiated carcinoma, lipoma, and mast cell tumor. Squamous cell carcinoma and lymphoma are the most common tumors of the larynx in the cat, but adenocarcinoma and other poorly differentiated round cell tumors have also been reported.[29]

Small lesions can be resected by mucosal resection or partial laryngectomy through an oral approach or ventral laryngotomy. Aggressive surgical intervention involves complete laryngectomy with permanent tracheostomy but has been reported only in isolated cases. Radioresponsive tumors can be treated with radiation therapy. Otherwise most treatment is palliative, consisting of airflow bypass of the laryngeal area through a permanent tracheostomy.

Prognosis for laryngeal tumors is guarded because most cases are quite advanced at the time of diagnosis. There are only isolated reports of management of canine and feline laryngeal tumors. Treatment of 4 cats with laryngeal squamous cell carcinoma with tube tracheostomy alone resulted in a median survival of only 3 days; chemotherapeutic treatment of 5 cats with varying types of laryngeal masses resulted in a median survival of 141 days.[38] Two cats with laryngeal lymphoma were treated with chemotherapy resulting in survival times of 60 and 1440 days.[29] In this same study, one cat with laryngeal squamous cell carcinoma was treated with prednisolone and had a survival time of 180 days.

A recent study reported on the placement of permanent tracheostomies in 5 cats with laryngeal carcinoma.[39] Survival at home ranged from 2 to 281 days with 2 cats dying from tracheostomy site occlusion and 3 cats euthanized because of disease progression.

Benign Growths

Inflammatory laryngeal disease is an uncommon nonneoplastic condition of the arytenoid cartilages of the larynx that has been reported in both dogs and cats. It can be granulomatous, lymphocytic-plasmacytic, or eosinophilic in nature, with multiple factors likely contributing to the development of the disease. Severe cases can result in laryngeal stenosis and significant upper airway obstruction. Biopsy of the mass is crucial to differentiate this disease from neoplasia, although it is still possible that inflammatory changes can represent a secondary response to underlying neoplasia. Treatment of inflammatory laryngeal disease is palliative and consists of debulking the mass, steroid therapy, or permanent tracheostomy. Permanent tracheostomy has been associated with a higher mortality in cats with inflammatory laryngeal disease than in cats undergoing permanent tracheostomy for any other reason.[40]

Benign laryngeal cysts also have been described in isolated cases.[41,42] Cysts are typically epithelial in origin and stem from the ventral aspect of the larynx. Surgical removal is usually curative.

SUMMARY

Diseases of the larynx can lead to life-threatening upper airway obstruction. Fundamental knowledge of laryngeal anatomy and use of appropriate sedation or anesthetic protocols are essential for thorough assessment of laryngeal structure and function. Prognosis is variable depending on the underlying cause.

REFERENCES

1. Monnet E, Tobias KM. Larynx. In: Tobias KM, Johnston SA, editors. Veterinary surgery small animal. St Louis (MO): Elsevier; 2012. p. 1724.
2. Ridyard AE, Corcoran BM, Tasker S, et al. Spontaneous laryngeal paralysis in four white-coated German shepherd dogs. J Small Anim Pract 2000;41:558–61.
3. Venker-van Haagen AJ, Bouw J, Hartman W. Hereditary transmission of laryngeal paralysis in bouviers. J Am Anim Hosp Assoc 1981;18:75–6.
4. O'Brien JA, Hendriks J. Inherited laryngeal paralysis. Analysis in the husky cross. Vet Q 1986;8:301–2.
5. Polizopoulou ZS, Koutinas AF, Papadopoulos GC, et al. Juvenile laryngeal paralysis in three Siberian husky x Alaskan malamute puppies. Vet Rec 2003;153: 624–7.
6. Braund KG, Shores A, Cochrane S, et al. Laryngeal paralysis-polyneuropathy complex in young Dalmatians. Am J Vet Res 1994;55:534–42.
7. Mahony OM, Knowles KE, Braund KG, et al. Laryngeal paralysis-polyneuropathy complex in young Rottweilers. J Vet Intern Med 1998;12:330–7.
8. Shelton GD, Podell M, Poncelet L, et al. Inherited polyneuropathy in Leonberger dogs: a mixed or intermediate form of Charcot-Marie-Tooth disease? Muscle Nerve 2003;27:471–7.
9. Gabriel A, Poncelet L, Van Ham L, et al. Laryngeal paralysis-polyneuropathy complex in young related Pyrenean mountain dogs. J Small Anim Pract 2006;47:144–9.
10. Stanley BJ, Hauptman JG, Fritz MC, et al. Esophageal dysfunction in dogs with idiopathic laryngeal paralysis: a controlled cohort study. Vet Surg 2010;39: 139–49.
11. Thieman KM, Krahwinkel DJ, Sims MH, et al. Histopathological confirmation of polyneuropathy in 11 dogs with laryngeal paralysis. J Am Anim Hosp Assoc 2010;46:161–7.
12. Jaggy A, Oliver JE, Ferguson DC, et al. Neurological manifestations of hypothyroidism: a retrospective study of 29 dogs. J Vet Intern Med 1994;8:328–36.
13. MacPhail CM, Monnet E. Outcome of and postoperative complications in dogs undergoing surgical treatment of laryngeal paralysis: 140 cases (1985–1998). J Am Vet Med Assoc 2001;218:1949–56.
14. Rudorf H, Barr FJ, Lane JG. The role of ultrasound in the assessment of laryngeal paralysis in the dog. Vet Radiol Ultrasound 2001;42:338–43.
15. Stadler K, Hartman S, Matheson J, et al. Computed tomographic imaging of dogs with primary laryngeal or tracheal airway obstruction. Vet Radiol Ultrasound 2011; 52:377–84.

16. Radlinsky MG, Williams J, Frank PM, et al. Comparison of three clinical techniques for the diagnosis of laryngeal paralysis in dogs. Vet Surg 2009;38:434–8.

17. Jackson AM, Tobias K, Long C, et al. Effects of various anesthetic agents on laryngeal motion during laryngoscopy in normal dogs. Vet Surg 2004;33:102–6.

18. Miller CJ, McKiernan BC, Pace J, et al. The effects of doxapram hydrochloride (Dopram-V) on laryngeal function in healthy dogs. J Vet Intern Med 2002;16: 524–8.

19. Tobias KM, Jackson AM, Harvey RC, et al. Effects of doxapram HCl on laryngeal function of normal dogs and dogs with naturally occurring laryngeal paralysis. Vet Anaesth Analg 2004;31:258–63.

20. Nicholson I, Baines S. Complications associated with temporary tracheostomy tubes in 42 dogs (1998 to 2007). J Small Anim Pract 2012;53:108–14.

21. Greenberg MJ, Bureau S, Monnet E. Effects of suture tension during unilateral cricoarytenoid lateralization on canine laryngeal resistance in vitro. Vet Surg 2007; 36:526–32.

22. Ross JT, Matthiesen DT, Noone KE, et al. Complications and long-term results after partial laryngectomy for the treatment of idiopathic laryngeal paralysis in 45 dogs. Vet Surg 1991;20:169–73.

23. Holt D, Harvey C. Idiopathic laryngeal paralysis: results of treatment by bilateral vocal fold resection in 40 dogs. J Am Anim Hosp Assoc 1994;30:389–95.

24. Zikes C, McCarthy T. Bilateral ventriculocordectomy via ventral laryngotomy for idiopathic laryngeal paralysis in 88 dogs. J Am Anim Hosp Assoc 2012;48: 234–44.

25. Schofield DM, Norris J, Sadanaga KK. Bilateral thyroarytenoid cartilage lateralization and vocal fold excision with mucosoplasty for treatment of idiopathic laryngeal paralysis: 67 dogs (1998–2005). Vet Surg 2007;36:519–25.

26. Olivieri M, Voghera SG, Fossum TW. Video-assisted left partial arytenoidectomy by diode laser photoablation for treatment of canine laryngeal paralysis. Vet Surg 2009;38:439–44.

27. Hammel SP, Hottinger HA, Novo RE. Postoperative results of unilateral arytenoid lateralization for treatment of idiopathic laryngeal paralysis in dogs: 39 cases (1996–2002). J Am Vet Med Assoc 2006;228:1215–20.

28. Weinstein J, Weisman D. Intraoperative evaluation of the larynx following unilateral arytenoid lateralization for acquired idiopathic laryngeal paralysis in dogs. J Am Anim Hosp Assoc 2010;46:241–8.

29. Taylor SS, Harvey AM, Barr FJ, et al. Laryngeal disease in cats: a retrospective study of 35 cases. J Feline Med Surg 2009;11:954–62.

30. Hardie RJ, Gunby J, Bjorling DE. Arytenoid lateralization for treatment of laryngeal paralysis in 10 cats. Vet Surg 2009;38:445–51.

31. Thunberg B, Lantz GC. Evaluation of unilateral arytenoid lateralization for the treatment of laryngeal paralysis in 14 cats. J Am Anim Hosp Assoc 2010;46: 418–24.

32. Rudorf H, Barr F. Echolaryngography in cats. Vet Radiol Ultrasound 2002;43(4): 353–7.

33. Pink JJ, Doyle RS, Hughes JM, et al. Laryngeal collapse in seven brachycephalic puppies. J Small Anim Pract 2006;47:131–5.

34. Lorison D, Bright RM, White RA. Brachycephalic airway obstruction syndrome—a review of 118 cases. Canine Pract 1997;22:18–21.

35. Poncet CM, Dupre GP, Freiche VG, et al. Long-term results of upper respiratory syndrome surgery and gastrointestinal tract medical treatment in 51 brachycephalic dogs. J Small Anim Pract 2006;47:137–42.

36. Torrez CV, Hunt GB. Results of surgical correction of abnormalities associated with brachycephalic airway obstruction syndrome in dogs in Australia. J Small Anim Pract 2006;47:150–4.

37. White RN. Surgical management of laryngeal collapse associated with brachycephalic airway obstruction syndrome in dogs. J Small Anim Pract 2012;53:44–50.

38. Jakubiak MJ, Siedlecki CT, Zenger E, et al. Laryngeal, laryngotracheal, and tracheal masses in cats: 27 cats (1998-2003). J Am Anim Hosp Assoc 2005; 41:310–6.

39. Guenther-Yenke CL, Rozanski EA. Tracheostomy in cats: 23 cases (1998-2006). J Feline Med Surg 2007;9(6):451–7.

40. Stepnik MW, Mehl ML, Hardie EM, et al. Outcome of permanent tracheostomy for treatment of upper airway obstruction in cats: 21 cases (1990-2007). J Am Vet Med Assoc 2009;234:638–43.

41. Rudorf H, Lane JG, Brown PJ, et al. Ultrasonographic diagnosis of a laryngeal cyst in a cat. J Small Anim Pract 1999;40:275–7.

42. Cuddy LC, Bacon NJ, Coomer AR, et al. Excision of a congenital laryngeal cyst in a five-month-old dog via a lateral extraluminal approach. J Am Vet Med Assoc 2010;236:1328–33.

Chronic Rhinitis in the Cat

Nicki Reed, BVM&S, Cert VR, DSAM (Feline), MRCVS

KEYWORDS

- Feline chronic rhinitis • Nasal biopsy • Neutrophilic inflammation • Herpesvirus
- Bacteria • Treatment

KEY POINTS

- Feline chronic rhinitis and/or rhinosinusitis is the second most common cause of feline rhinitis, accounting for approximately 35% of cases.
- Proposed causes relate to initial turbinate damage by feline herpesvirus-1 likely combined with an impaired or deranged immune response, allowing establishment of recurring secondary bacterial infections.
- Bacteria commonly identified are typically commensal to the oropharynx; the role of *Bordetella bronchiseptica* and *Mycoplasma* spp as primary agents is unclear at this time.
- Repeated short courses of antibacterials may result in selection for *Pseudomonas* spp.
- Treatment is primarily supportive, comprising antibacterials, mucolytics or decongestants, antiviral therapies, and in severe cases surgery. Nasal flushing to remove mucus is often beneficial.
- Owners need to be counseled that cure is unlikely. Treatment aims to reduce the frequency and severity of episodes.

INTRODUCTION

Feline chronic rhinitis can be defined as inflammation of the nasal cavity that has been present for 4 weeks or longer, either intermittently or continuously.[1] Because the frontal sinuses can also be involved, the condition may be called chronic rhinosinusitis (CRS). The diagnosis accounts for approximately 35% of cases of feline rhinitis[2,3] and, after neoplasia, is the second most common cause of chronic nasal discharge in cats.[3] Despite being a relatively common condition in feline practice, it can be a frustrating disease to manage.

CAUSES

It has been proposed that primary viral infection, especially by feline herpesvirus-1 (FHV-1), causes damage to the mucosal epithelium and underlying turbinate

---

Disclosures: The author declares no funding sources or conflicts of interest.
The Hospital for Small Animals, Easter Bush Veterinary Centre, The University of Edinburgh, Roslin, Midlothian EH25 9RG, Scotland, UK
E-mail address: nreed1@staffmail.ed.ac.uk

bones, thereby predisposing to recurrent bacterial rhinitis.[4–6] One study used a polymerase chain reaction (PCR) technique to identify FHV-1 DNA in nasal biopsy samples but failed to show a difference in isolation rates between cats with CRS and healthy control cats.[6] This suggests that recrudescence of viral disease per se may be less important in the role of CRS than other factors such as structural damage, secondary bacterial infection and impaired immune function.[7–10]

Although bacterial infection has been identified in 69% to 90% of cases,[1,6] primary bacterial infection is considered rare. Mixed growth of commensal organisms is frequently identified; more significance might be attached to a heavy pure growth of one organism, especially those that are considered pathogenic (**Box 1**).[6] Rarer bacteria isolated from cases of CRS include *Haemophilus* spp[11] and *Capnocytophaga* spp.[12]

One study[10] attempted to evaluate the role of *Bartonella* spp in CRS but failed to identify these organisms by culture of blood samples or PCR of nasal biopsies, with the exception of one case that had a nasopharyngeal abscess. Serologic testing did not identify differences in seropositivity to *Bartonella* spp between cats with CRS and three control groups. Although the study was underpowered, it did not support a role for these organisms in CRS.

The role of *Mycoplasma* spp in rhinitis remains uncertain because these organisms have been considered part of the commensal flora in the upper respiratory tract. *Mycoplasma* spp were detected in cats affected by CRS but not in control cats, suggesting that they may play a role in this disease complex.[6] Use of PCR may facilitate identification of *Mycoplasma* spp, which can be difficult to culture.[13]

Retroviral infection was previously suggested to be associated with CRS[14] because in one study 55% of cats were positive for feline leukemia (FeLV) infection.[15] However, subsequent studies showed a reduced prevalence of retroviral infection (0%–7%).[1,16,17] This mirrored the declining prevalence of infection in the feline population after the introduction of FeLV vaccination.

Box 1
Potentially pathogenic bacteria in feline CRS
Pseudomonas aeruginosa
Escherichia coli
Streptococcus viridans
Staphylococcus pseudintermedius
Pasteurella multocida
Corynebacterium spp
Actinomyces spp
Bordetella bronchiseptica
Mycoplasma spp
All anaerobes
Data from Johnson LR, Foley JE, De Cock HE, et al. Assessment of infectious organisms associated with chronic rhinosinusitis in cats. J Am Vet Med Assoc 2005;227(4):583.

PATIENT HISTORY

Chronic rhinitis is often found in cats with some or all of the following history:

- Usually identified in young to middle-aged cats although there is a wide age range affected (0.5–16 years)[3,10]
- Might have had a history of "cat flu" as a kitten although this is often difficult to establish
- Recurrent episodes of nasal discharge (**Fig. 1**) that can be
  - Serous (initially)
  - Mucoid
  - Mucopurulent
  - Sanguineous (less common)
  - Unilateral, bilateral or unilateral progressing to bilateral
- Sneezing
- Stertorous respiration
- Episodes may be associated with stressors such as boarding, breeding or neutering
- Cats can become inappetent at times of clinical signs due to
  - Inability to smell food
  - Difficulty breathing
  - Pyrexia
- Episodes often respond to antibacterials but relapse is common
- Gagging, choking, or reverse sneezing is more commonly seen with nasopharyngeal diseases but could be observed with accumulation of discharges in the nasopharynx.

PHYSICAL EXAMINATION

In addition to a complete physical examination, particular attention should be made to examining the specific features listed in **Table 1**. To perform a thorough oral examination, general anesthesia is invariably required.

DIAGNOSTIC TESTING

The diagnosis of CRS is usually based on excluding other conditions that could cause signs of upper respiratory tract disease. Differential diagnoses to consider for the

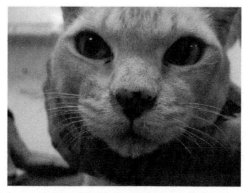

Fig. 1. Cat with CRS demonstrating bilateral serous nasal discharge.

Table 1
Salient features of physical examination in CRS

Assessment	Significance
Nasal airflow Can be assessed by observing condensation on a cold microscope slide, or holding wisps of cotton wool in front of nares	Decreased nasal airflow is often due to obstruction with mass lesions (neoplastic, fungal, or foreign body related)
Presence of nasal discharge Unilateral or bilateral; nature	Unilateral discharge is more common with foreign body or neoplasia than CRS Discharge is typically mucoid, becoming mucopurulent with secondary bacterial infection
Facial symmetry	Facial asymmetry is more commonly seen with neoplasia or fungal infection, but can be seen with CRS
Facial pain May be appreciated on palpation or if the cat demonstrates head aversion when approached	Can be seen with CRS, neoplasia, fungal infections, foreign bodies, or dental disease, and indicates that analgesia should be provided
Conjunctivitis	Can indicate infection with certain organisms such as FHV-1, FCV, *Chlamydophila felis*, or *Mycoplasma* spp that may or may not be related to rhinitis
Epiphora Fluorescein staining can be used to assess patency of nasolacrimal duct	May have concurrent keratitis or ocular ulceration Chronic inflammation can cause blockage of the nasolacrimal system
Retinal examination	Can identify chorioretinitis associated with cryptococcal infection or lymphoma
Oral examination	Used to identify cleft palate, oronasal fistula, mass lesions causing ventral deviation of the soft palate Visualization of the nasopharynx can be facilitated by retracting the soft palate with a spay hook and using a dental mirror
Otic examination	Mass lesions or bowing of the tympanic membrane can be seen in association with nasopharyngeal polyps
Lymph node palpation The submandibular and retropharyngeal lymph nodes should be evaluated	Lymph node enlargement is a nonspecific finding, although asymmetry can suggest disease such as neoplasia, fungal infection, or foreign body is more likely than CRS

clinical presentation of sneezing and nasal discharge are given in **Box 2**. To eliminate these other conditions, several tests are generally required. Investigations typically progress from the least invasive to the most invasive.

Laboratory Analysis

Routine hematology, biochemistry, and urinalysis findings are nonspecific but give information about the general health of the cat before administration of general anesthesia or therapeutics. Retroviral testing does not assist with the diagnosis but contributes toward the overall health status of the cat and may have an effect on prognosis.

Box 2
Differential diagnoses for chronic sneezing and nasal discharge

Neoplasia (lymphoma, adenocarcinoma, sarcoma)

Nasopharyngeal polyp

Foreign body

Fungal infection (*Crytpococcus* spp, *Aspergillus* spp, *Penicillium* spp)

Allergic rhinitis

Nasopharyngeal stenosis

Trauma

Congenital (cleft palate; extreme brachycephalic conformation)

Dental disease (oronasal fistula; tooth root infection or abscess)

Inflammatory polyps of the nasal turbinates (mesenchymal nasal hamartoma)

Serologic evaluation for respiratory viruses is of no use due to the high prevalence of seropositivity in healthy cats.[18] In cases in which *Cryptococcus* infection is suspected, performance of a latex cryptococcal antigen test is useful for both diagnosis and monitoring.[19] See elsewhere in this issue for further information on feline aspergillosis by Barrs and Talbot.

Oropharyngeal and Conjunctival Swabbing

In cats with acute upper respiratory tract disease, oropharyngeal and conjunctival swabs can be submitted for bacterial culture (*Chlamydophila felis, Bordetella bronchiseptica, Mycoplasma* spp), virus isolation (FHV-1, feline calicivirus [FCV]), and PCR (FHV-1, FCV, *C felis, B bronchiseptica*, and *Mycoplasma* spp). Special transport media is required, particularly for virus isolation. Interpretation of results can be problematic. A negative result does not necessarily exclude the infection as the cause of the disease, particularly with fragile organisms that are difficult to culture (eg, *Mycoplasma*) or if the organism is intermittently shed (eg, FHV-1). Conversely, identifying FHV-1 or FCV does not always explain the clinical signs, due to the high prevalence of these infections in the healthy cat population and inability to differentiate positive test results from presence of vaccinal strains.[20–22]

Nasal Swabbing

Swabbing nasal discharge for culture is of minimal benefit because it is likely that only commensal bacteria of the oropharynx will be cultured.[23] Cytology is likely to reveal degenerate neutrophils as the predominant cell type and, although bacteria may be identified, their significance is questionable. The finding of encapsulated yeast organisms would be supportive of *Cryptococcus* infection; use of Romanowsky stains, new methylene blue, or Gram stain enables the organism to be seen surrounded by a clear halo.[24]

Special Considerations for Epistaxis

If frank hemorrhage from the nose is part of the presenting complaint, a coagulation panel should be assessed in addition to a platelet count. If the nasal discharge is sanguineous in nature, if the cat is older than 8 years old, or if concurrent kidney disease is identified, systolic blood pressure should also be measured.

Diagnostic Imaging

Accurate positioning requires general anesthesia, and several radiographic views should be taken to fully evaluate the nasal cavity and sinuses.[25] Superimposition of the mandible in the dorsoventral views necessitates use of dental film or performance of a ventral 30° rostral-dorsocaudal view.[25] Radiological interpretation is given elsewhere[26]; however, findings consistent with CRS include unilateral or bilateral soft-tissue and/or fluid opacification of the nasal cavity and/or frontal sinuses with blurring of turbinate structures. Erosion of the turbinate bones and mass lesions can be identified radiographically in cats with neoplasia or chronic rhinitis,[27] making a definitive diagnosis by radiological assessment impossible.

CT is considered superior to radiography for imaging the nasal cavity and paranasal sinuses in dogs[28–30] and the same is likely true in the cat. The CT appearance of the normal feline nasal cavity and paranasal sinuses has been described.[31] Studies comparing the CT appearance of nasal neoplasia and inflammatory disease in cats identified that many imaging findings overlapped between these conditions (**Fig. 2**).[32,33] Features occurring significantly more often in cats with neoplasia included lysis of the ventral aspect of the maxilla or vomer bone; unilateral lysis of the ethmoturbinates or dorsal and lateral aspects of the maxilla; bilateral lysis of the orbital lamina; and unilateral soft tissue opacification of the frontal sinus, sphenoid sinus, or retrobulbar space.[33]

Nasal Flush

Nasal flushes can be performed to collect diagnostic material; however, flushing may also be used as a therapeutic technique. The procedure should be performed under general anesthesia with a cuffed endotracheal tube in place. The cat is placed in sternal recumbency with the head angled down to facilitate drainage of fluid. Descriptions of diagnostic and therapeutic flushes follow:

- Diagnostic and therapeutic flushes may then be performed as follows: A 6 to 8F sterile catheter is inserted into the rostral nasal cavity (not beyond the level of the medial canthus of the eye). The nasopharynx is occluded by dorsal digital pressure on the soft palate. Next, 2 to 4 mL of sterile saline is gently flushed down the catheter followed by aspiration of the fluid to obtain a sample for aerobic and anaerobic culture (±fungal culture and PCR or *Mycoplasma* testing where indicated).

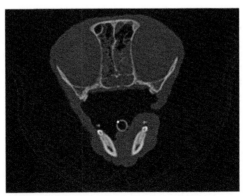

Fig. 2. CT scan of a cat with CRS demonstrating loss of turbinate structure and accumulation of fluid within the nasal cavity. Deviation of the septum can be a normal finding in cats.

- Therapeutic flush. The oropharynx is packed with a gauze swab to prevent aspiration of material and allow collection of any foreign material that is flushed from the nasal cavity. A 10 mL syringe is filled with sterile saline and the tip inserted into the nostril. The naris is compressed around the syringe tip and the contralateral naris occluded. The syringe is then depressed with steady pressure to force material caudally onto the swab (**Fig. 3**). The process is repeated until all the mucopurulent material is flushed through. Next, it is performed on the contralateral side. Mass lesions and foreign bodies can also be dislodged by this technique.

Although good agreement has been reported between bacterial cultures from nasal flush samples compared with biopsy samples,[6] discordant results were reported between these two methods in 32%, 10%, and 18% of cases when culture of aerobic, anaerobic, and *Mycoplasma* organisms, respectively, were considered.[34] The increased recovery of organisms from nasal flushes could be due to culture of superficial organisms not involved in the disease process. Alternatively, it could reflect increased difficulty in culturing representative bacteria from tissue samples because the flush fluid is directly inoculated onto culture media whereas, with biopsy material, maceration is required.[34]

Endoscopy

The nasopharynx can be evaluated with a flexible endoscope (eg, 3–5 mm bronchoscope) capable of 180° flexion. Endoscopic evaluation of the nasal cavity can be performed in a normograde fashion using either a rigid endoscope with a viewing angle of 0° to 30° or a flexible endoscope of 2 to 3 mm diameter. Saline flushing via the biopsy channel can remove mucus and facilitate visualization of the mucosa. A throat pack or swabs should be placed in the pharynx to prevent aspiration of material. The nasal mucosa overlying the turbinates should appear pink and smooth and the vessels should be clearly seen. Abnormalities seen with chronic rhinitis include congestion and decreased visibility of the capillaries, hyperemia, increased fragility, ulceration, and increased mucus. In addition, turbinate destruction can give rise to increased space when trying to navigate the meatus.

Endoscopy allows collection of targeted cytology or biopsy samples. Evaluation of the frontal sinuses cannot normally be undertaken in cats, although extensive turbinate destruction from fungal infection permitted passage of a bronchoscope in one case.[35]

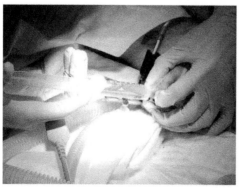

Fig. 3. A nasal flush being performed to remove mucus and potentially foreign bodies.

Brush Cytology

An endoscopic cytology brush can be passed down the biopsy channel or passed adjacent to the endoscope to allow direct visualization[2]; however, samples can be nondiagnostic due to poor cellularity.[2,36] Comparison between cytologic and histologic samples has shown poor agreement, with only 25% of samples having the same predominant cell type.[2] Neoplasia was incorrectly diagnosed as inflammatory in 27% of cases.[36] Because histopathology is likely to give a more accurate diagnosis, this technique is rarely used.

Nasal Biopsy

Before taking nasal biopsy samples, the author recommends evaluation of coagulation status. As a minimum, prothrombin time, activated partial thromboplastin time, and fibrinogen should be measured. However, performance of a buccal mucosal bleeding time also allows assessment of function of platelets and von Willebrand factor. Samples can be obtained via the biopsy channel of the endoscope; however, biopsy samples obtained are very small. Targeted sampling of focal lesions can also be achieved by passing the biopsy instrument alongside the rigid telescope or, for diffuse disease, blind biopsies can be diagnostic. These can be performed with 3 mm biopsy cups (**Fig. 4**) and both right and left nasal cavities should be biopsied. The nasopharynx can also be biopsied via the biopsy channel of a flexible endoscope.

Where endoscopic equipment is not available, a suction biopsy can be obtained with a plastic catheter, the tip of which has been angled to 45° and suction applied with a 10 to 20 mL syringe.[37] Biopsy material should be submitted in plain tubes for bacterial and fungal culture as well as fixed in formalin for histopathology.

Inflammatory infiltrate is classified according to the predominant cell type and is often described as lymphoplasmacytic, neutrophilic (suppurative), or mixed.[2,6] Neutrophilic infiltrate seems to be twice as common as lymphoplasmacytic infiltrate[2,17,38] and associated with more severe inflammatory changes.[38] Although neutrophilic infiltrate has been classified as acute rhinitis by some investigators,[3] and lymphoplasmacytic infiltrate considered the most common form of chronic rhinitis by others,[39] these differences may simply reflect the spectrum of one disease. The nature of the inflammatory infiltrate might depend on the presence or absence of bacterial infection at the time of sampling because many cats with neutrophilic infiltrate have a chronic rather than acute history.

Other features that can be identified on histopathology include epithelial ulceration, fibrosis, turbinate destruction or remodeling, necrosis, and glandular hyperplasia.[40] The poor correlation between rhinoscopic appearance and histopathology indicates the need to obtain biopsy material bilaterally for histopathology.[38] Eosinophilic

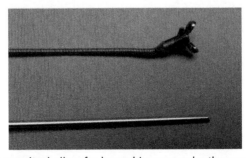

Fig. 4. 3 mm biopsy cups (*top*) allow for larger biopsy samples than can be obtained alongside a rigid endoscope (*bottom*).

infiltrate could suggest an allergic or parasitic origin, although this is unproven. Eosinophilic infiltrate in nasal biopsies from cats with rhinitis and concurrent signs of asthma has been identified on occasion by this author, as well as in a study of nasal histology in cats with experimentally induced allergic asthma,[41] which could support a role of allergy in eosinophilic rhinitis.

TREATMENT

Treatment of feline CRS is frustrating. No definitive therapy exists. Treatment is aimed at controlling episodes of clinical signs and preventing extension of disease. Owners need to be counseled regarding the recurrent nature of this condition and that treatment will not be curative. Multimodal therapy can be used to address different aspects of the disease.

Antibacterials

Ideally, choice of antibacterial agent should be based on culture and sensitivity results from nasal biopsies and/or nasal flush fluid.[6] Due to the recurrent nature of this disease, however, owners may be unwilling to subject the cat to repeated general anesthesia every time there is recurrence of clinical signs. As such, empiric prescribing often has to be used, with the choice of antibiotic based on the spectrum of infectious agents typically identified (see **Box 1**). In addition, the antibacterial chosen should have good penetration to bone and cartilage. Suggested antibacterial choices are given in **Table 2**. Due to the chronic, deep nature of these infections, this author normally prescribes therapy for a 6 to 8 week period.

Although a few studies have assessed the efficacy of antibacterials in the treatment of acute rhinitis and *Chlamydophila* infections,[42–47] these studies are based on culture of superficial ocular, nasal, or oropharyngeal swabs. *Pseudomonas* spp were not identified in these studies, yet this is a commonly identified organism when deeper nasal samples are obtained.[6,8] *Pseudomonas* spp are resistant to the commonly used antibacterials listed in **Table 2**; therefore, repeated antibacterial courses that eliminate other commensal organisms are likely to contribute to selection for this organism. Culture can identify appropriate sensitivity to veterinary-licensed antibacterials such as marbofloxacin or pradofloxacin. Alternatively, a licensed human antibacterial, such as a third-generation cephalosporin (eg, ceftazidime, cefoperazone) or aminoglycoside (eg, amikacin, tobramycin), might be required, although due consideration must be given to renal and ototoxicity with the aminoglycosides.[48] Efficacy of antibacterials might be enhanced by the supportive therapies discussed below.

Improvement to Air Flow

Nasal flushing

The presence of tenacious mucopurulent discharge within the nasal cavity can not only result in difficulty breathing but may also occlude the ostia, impairing drainage of fluid from the frontal sinuses. This, in turn, results in sinusitis, which can cause frontal sinus pain, contributing to lethargy and inappetence. Periodic nasal flushing as described above may provide clinical relief by removing this mucopurulent material.

Nebulization

Nebulization involves suspension of droplets of a liquid (usually saline) within a propellant gas (usually air or oxygen) (**Fig. 5**). Smaller droplets (0.5–5.0 μm) are deposited within the lower airways, whereas larger droplets (20.0 μm) are deposited within the nasopharynx.[49] Although there are no studies demonstrating efficacy, nebulization could be beneficial in making secretions less viscous and promoting ciliary clearance.

Table 2
Oral antibacterial drugs used for management of CRS

Antibacterial	Spectrum	Dosage	Comments
Amoxicillin-clavulanate	Staphylococci Streptococci Chlamydophila E coli Pasteurella Bordetella Anaerobes	10–20 mg/kg q 8 h	Not effective against Pseudomonas
Azithromycin	Staphylococci Streptococci Chlamydophila Mycoplasma Bordetella Anaerobes	10–15 mg/kg q 24 h	Inconsistent efficacy against Chlamydophila[43] Not effective against Pseudomonas
Chloramphenicol	Staphylococci Streptococci Chlamydophila E coli Bordetella Anaerobes	20–40 mg/kg q 12 h	Can be ineffective, or resistance can develop with Pseudomonas Monitor hematology weekly due to risk of myelosuppression
Clindamycin	Staphylococci Streptococci Chlamydophila Actinomyces Anaerobes Mycoplasma, variable efficacy	10–12 mg/kg q 12–24 h	Not effective against Pseudomonas or other gram- negative organisms Can cause esophagitis and esophageal strictures
Doxycycline	Chlamydophila Pasteurella Bordetella Mycoplasma Actinomyces	10 mg/kg q 24 h	Good penetration into frontal sinuses Not effective against Pseudomonas or E coli Only effective against a few Staphylococci and Streptococci spp Can cause esophagitis and esophageal strictures May also have an immunomodulatory effect
Marbofloxacin	Staphylococci Streptococci E coli Pasteurella Mycoplasma (Pseudomonas)	2 mg/kg q 24 h	Could be less likely to cause retinal toxicity than enrofloxacin Pseudomonas may develop resistance
Metronidazole	Anaerobes	15–20 mg/kg q 12 h	Unpalatable Narrow spectrum, typically combined with other drugs
Pradofloxacin	Staphylococci Streptococci E coli Pasteurella Mycoplasma (Pseudomonas)	5–10 mg/kg q 24 h[46]	Greater activity against anaerobes than other quinolones Less likely to cause retinal toxicity than enrofloxacin Pseudomonas may develop resistance

Data from Greene CE, Calpin J. Antimicrobial drug formulary. In: Greene CE, editor. Infectious diseases of the dog and cat. 4th edition. St Louis (MO): Elsevier Saunders; 2012. p. 1207–320; and Plumb DC. Plumb's veterinary drug handbook. 6th edition. Ames (IA): Blackwell Publishing Professional; 2008.

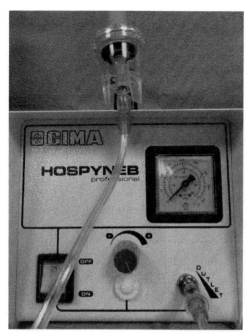

Fig. 5. A hospital nebulizer can be used to humidify the upper airways and facilitate removal of nasal discharges.

A suggested regime is 15 minutes every 8 to 12 hours. Nebulization can also be used to deliver antibacterial agents topically (primarily aminoglycosides). Inhaled N-acetyl-cysteine may cause bronchospasm and epithelial toxicity, attributed to its hypertonic-ity[50]; therefore although advocated by some, it is not recommended by this author. If nebulization is not available, instillation of saline drops can improve hydration of the nasal passages. This therapeutic modality does not seem particularly well toler-ated by cats; therefore, placing the cat in a steamy environment (eg, shower room) is an alternate option, although use of a standard humidifier is more likely to be beneficial.

Mucolytics
Mucolytics such as bromhexine can be considered. Their primary action is to facilitate mucociliary clearance within the tracheobronchial tree; therefore, their role in sino-nasal disease is unknown (**Table 3**).

Decongestants
Decongestants might improve nasal airflow by reducing mucosal edema through vasoconstriction (see **Table 3**). Unfortunately this is often followed by rebound vaso-dilation and worsening signs; therefore, it is recommended that topical use of these drugs is limited to 3 days.[39] As with mucolytics, there is no published evidence of benefit in the management of CRS.

Antivirals

The rationale for using antiviral therapy is based on the presumed association between recrudescence of chronic FHV-1 infection and episodes of clinical signs. The lack of

Table 3
Mucolytics and decongestants for clinical management of CRS

Drug	Dosage	Comment
Bromhexine (Bisolvon)	3 mg/cat IM q 24 h 1 mg/kg po q 24 h	Bronchial secretolytic
Dimenhydrinate (Dramamine)	4 mg/cat po q 8 h	Antihistamine, antiemetic, anticholinergic Latter contributes to decongestant effect
Ephedrine hydrochloride (0.5% nasal drops)	1 drop each nostril q 12–24 h	Only administer for 72 h to avoid rebound congestion
Oxymetazoline (Afrazin; Afrin)	1 drop each nostril q 12 h 1 drop each nostril q 24 h	Maximum 48 h Maximum 72 h
Phenylephrine hydrochloride (2.5% ophthalmic solution; Little Noses)	1 drop each nostril q 24 h	Maximum 72 h
Pseudoephedrine (Sudafed; Galpseud)	1 mg/kg po q 8 h	Administration facilitated by use of 6 mg/mL syrup rather than tablets
Xylometazoline (Otrovine; Otradrops)	1 drop each nostril q 24 h	Maximum 72 h

Data from Refs.[39,51–53]

evidence to support current active infection with FHV-1 in association with signs of rhinitis likely accounts for the weak evidence to support use of these treatments.

Interferon
Although FHV-1 is susceptible to interferon (IFN) in vitro, clinical trials have yet to demonstrate a clear benefit. Although IFN-α can be used topically for ocular lesions, systemic administration is more logical for respiratory disease hence feline recombinant IFN-ω is more appropriate for administration by this route. A suggested dosage is 1 MegaUnit/kg subcutaneously every 24 hours for 5 days.[54] No clear efficacy in feline rhinitis has been reported to date.

Famciclovir
Famciclovir is a prodrug of the deoxyguanosine analog penciclovir.[55] As such, it is virustatic rather than virucidal. Although controlled clinical trials have not been performed, improvement in clinical signs was reported in two cats with CRS.[56] The optimal dosage is not yet known. Dosages have varied from 62.5 mg/cat[56] every 24 hours to 90 mg/kg every 8 hours[57] with a protracted course (up to 4 months) appearing to be well tolerated.

Lysine
Lysine is thought to have an antiviral effect by competing for arginine, an essential amino acid for viral replication.[55] Studies have demonstrated decreased conjunctivitis and viral shedding in cats experimentally infected with FHV-1 that are treated with lysine.[58,59] Unfortunately, this has not translated into decreased clinical signs of upper respiratory tract disease in shelter cats administered oral lysine or lysine-supplemented diets.[60–62] Although no clinical benefit has been proven in the shelter situation, client-owned cats are likely subjected to less stress than shelter cats, and it could be of use in this population, provided the stress of administering the drug does not outweigh any benefit. The recommended dosage is 500 mg/cat twice daily.[55]

Antihistamines

Some investigators have proposed that antihistamines are beneficial[39,53]; however, they could have the unwanted side effect of further drying out inspissated secretions. The nature of the cellular infiltrate might guide the decision to use antihistamines, which could be more beneficial with an eosinophilic or possibly lymphoplasmacytic infiltrate than with a neutrophilic or suppurative infiltrate. The individual response to antihistamines is variable; therefore, it can be beneficial to try different classes of antihistamine before deciding they are of no benefit (**Table 4**).

Antiinflammatories

Johnson and colleagues[63] identified increased levels of gene transcription for the inflammatory cytokines interleukin (IL)-6, IL-10, IL-12 p40, IFN-γ, and RANTES in nasal biopsies with an inflammatory infiltrate compared with normal biopsies. There was no alteration in gene transcription of Il-4, IL-5, IL-16, and IL-18. This indicates a predominant helper T cell (Th)1 response to inflammatory stimuli, which could lead to more targeted therapies to modify this inflammatory response.

Glucocorticoids

Glucocorticoids have several effects on the immune system, and they could be considered beneficial in CRS because they reduce mucosal edema and migration of inflammatory cells. However, there are no studies demonstrating benefit in cats with CRS, and they could potentially be detrimental in the presence of bacterial infection and a suppurative infiltrate. In addition, they could initiate recrudescence of herpes virus infection. Glucocorticoids can be administered orally or by inhalational therapy. If the latter route is used it is likely to be more effective if mucus build-up has been cleared first (eg, by nasal flushing or nebulization).

Nonsteroidal antiinflammatory drugs

Nonsteroidal antiinflammatory drugs (NSAIDs) might reduce sinus pain associated with CRS, thereby improving appetite and demeanor. There are no studies assessing the efficacy of the antiinflammatory effect, and they should not be considered in cats that are not well hydrated or in cats with renal insufficiency.

Leukotriene inhibitors

Leukotrienes are produced from arachidonic acid through the action of 5-lipoxygenase. They exert a chemoattractant effect on inflammatory cells, contributing to nasal

---

Table 4
Antihistamine options for CRS

Antihistamine Class	Drug	Dosage (Oral)
Alkylamine	Chlorpheniramine; chlorphenamine (Piriton; Chlor-Trimeton)	1–2 mg/cat q 8–12 h
Ethanolamine	Diphenhydramine (Nytol; Benadryl) Clemastine (Tavist-D; Tavegil)	2–4 mg/kg q 8 h 0.05–0.1 mg/kg q 12 h
Piperazine	Cetirizine Hydroxyzine (Atarax; Vistaril)	5 mg/cat q 12 h 2 mg/kg q 8–12 h
Piperidine	Loratidine (Claritin) Fexofenadine (Telfast)	0.5 mg/kg q 24 h 10 mg/cat q 12 h
Phenothiazine	Trimeprazine; alimemazine	0.5–1.0 mg/kg q 8–12 h
Antiserotonergic	Cyproheptadine (Periactin)	1 mg/cat q 12 h

Data from Refs.[39,51–53]

edema, increased vascular permeability, and mucus production. Levels of leukotri-enes can be reduced through blockade of 5-lipoxygenase (zileuton), thereby inhibiting production. Alternatively, the action of leukotrienes can be inhibited through blockade of the cysteinyl-leukotriene–1 receptor (zafirlukast, montelukast). Although leukotriene inhibition has been shown to be beneficial in humans with chronic rhinitis (particularly allergic rhinitis, concurrent nasal polyps, or aspirin intolerance),[64] the benefit in cats is unknown.

Immunomodulation

One study attempted to demonstrate immunomodulation of the inflammatory response following intraperitoneal injection of liposome-IL-2 DNA complexes to stim-ulate the innate immune response.[8] This demonstrated a reduction in sneezing in older cats with chronic rhinitis and a progressive decrease in TNFα mRNA expression; how-ever, the clinical utility of this experimental treatment is uncertain at this time.

Surgery

Surgical intervention in the management of CRS has been described.[16,65,66] Turbinec-tomy can be performed via a dorsal or ventral approach, and the latter is promoted as being more cosmetically acceptable to owners.[65,66] A procedure that allows debride-ment of chronically infected material from the frontal sinuses is likely beneficial over turbinectomy alone. Following stripping of affected periosteum, the ablated sinus can be packed with an autogenous fat graft,[16] polymethyl methacrylate bone cement (PMMA),[66] or PMMA infused with gentamicin.[66] Although good outcomes were re-ported, with compete resolution of signs in four of six cases,[16] and good-to-excellent outcome in nine of nineteen cases,[66] no comparison was made with medical management in the studies. Complications of surgery reported included failure to remove all the periosteal lining, surgical site abscessation, ataxia, death, and on-going nasal discharge.[16,66]

PROGNOSIS

The prognosis for CRS should be considered guarded. The condition is rarely cured, which can result in cats being euthanized if owners cannot cope with the expense of on-going treatment or the presence of persistent nasal discharge. There is the poten-tial for persistent inflammation to lead to development of nasal or nasopharyngeal polyps or nasopharyngeal stricture formation.[67,68] These structural abnormalities can also lead to the development of chronic rhinitis, therefore it can be difficult to eval-uate which condition came first. In addition, chronic obstruction of the eustachian tubes by purulent discharge can lead to otitis media. In some cases extensive bone lysis can occur, resulting in facial deformity or, potentially, erosion through the cribri-form plate and involvement of the brain.[69]

If owners are committed to administering medications and adjunct therapies, quality of life can be substantially improved, even though the condition is not cured. Surgical management can potentially affect a cure or a substantial improvement.

SUMMARY

Feline chronic rhinitis presents as recurring clinical signs of nasal discharge, sneezing, and stertor that can be accompanied by lethargy and inappetence. Diagnosis of this condition involves exclusion of other conditions that result in similar clinical signs and identification of an inflammatory infiltrate on nasal biopsy. Treatment is not curative and can involve prolonged courses of antibacterials in combination with adjunctive therapies and, in some cases, surgery. Prognosis is affected by owner commitment and can vary from excellent (surgery is curative) to poor (owners elect euthanasia).

REFERENCES

1. Cape L. Feline idiopathic chronic rhinosinusitis: a retrospective study of 30 cases. J Am Anim Hosp Assoc 1992;28(2):149–55.
2. Michiels L, Day MJ, Snaps F, et al. A retrospective study of non-specific rhinitis in 22 cats and the value of nasal cytology and histopathology. J Feline Med Surg 2003;5(5):279–85.
3. Henderson SM, Bradley K, Day MJ, et al. Investigation of nasal disease in the cat—a retrospective study of 77 cases. J Feline Med Surg 2004;6(4):245–57.
4. Ford RB. Pathogenesis and sequelae of feline viral respiratory infection. Supplement to Comp Cont Education Practice 1979;19(3):21–7.
5. Hawkins EC. Chronic viral upper respiratory disease in cats: differential diagnosis and management. Comp Cont Education Practice 1988;10(9):1003–12.
6. Johnson LR, Foley JE, De Cock HE, et al. Assessment of infectious organisms associated with chronic rhinosinusitis in cats. J Am Vet Med Assoc 2005; 227(4):579–85.
7. Johnson LR, Maggs DJ. Feline herpesvirus type-1 transcription is associated with increased nasal cytokine gene transcription in cats. Vet Microbiol 2005; 108(3–4):225–33.
8. Veir JK, Lappin MR, Dow SW. Evaluation of a novel immunotherapy for treatment of chronic rhinitis in cats. J Feline Med Surg 2006;8(6):400–11.
9. Gaskell R, Dawson S, Radford A, et al. Feline herpesvirus. Vet Res 2007;38(2): 337–54.
10. Berryessa NA, Johnson LR, Kasten RW, et al. Microbial culture of blood samples and serologic testing for bartonellosis in cats with chronic rhinosinusitis. J Am Vet Med Assoc 2008;233(7):1084–9.
11. Milner RJ, Horton JH, Crawford PC, et al. Suppurative rhinitis associated with *Haemophilus* species infection in a cat. J S Afr Vet Assoc 2004;75(2):103–7.
12. Frey E, Pressler B, Guy J, et al. *Capnocytophaga* sp isolated from a cat with chronic sinusitis and rhinitis. J Clin Microbiol 2003;41(11):5321–4.
13. Johnson LR, Drazenovich N, Foley JE. A comparison of routine culture with polymerase chain reaction technology for the detection of *Mycoplasma* species in feline nasal samples. J Vet Diagn Invest 2004;16(4):347–51.
14. Van Pelt DR, Lappin MR. Pathogenesis and treatment of feline rhinitis. Vet Clin North Am Small Anim Pract 1994;24(5):807–23.
15. Hardy WD. Feline leukemia virus non-neoplastic diseases. J Am Anim Hosp Assoc 1981;17(6):941–9.
16. Anderson GI. The treatment of chronic sinusitis in six cats by ethmoid conchal curettage and autogenous fat graft sinus ablation. Vet Surg 1987;16(2):131–4.
17. Demko JL, Cohn LA. Chronic nasal discharge in cats: 75 cases (1993-2004). J Am Vet Med Assoc 2007;230(7):1032–7.
18. Maggs DJ, Lappin MR, Reif JS, et al. Evaluation of serologic and viral detection methods for diagnosing feline herpesvirus-1 infection in cats with acute respiratory and chronic ocular disease. J Am Vet Med Assoc 1999;214(4):502–7.
19. Malik R, McPetrie R, Wigney DI, et al. A latex cryptococcal antigen agglutination test for diagnosis and monitoring of therapy for cryptococcosis. Aust Vet J 1996; 74(5):358–64.

20. Thiry E, Addie D, Belak S, et al. Feline herpesvirus infection: ABCD guidelines on prevention and management. J Feline Med Surg 2009;11(7):547–55.
21. Radford AD, Addie D, Belak S, et al. Feline calicivirus infection: ABCD guidelines on prevention and management. J Feline Med Surg 2009;11(7):556–64.
22. Maggs DJ, Clarke HE. Relative sensitivity of polymerase chain reaction assays used for detection of feline herpesvirus type 1 DNA in clinical samples and commercial vaccines. Am J Vet Res 2005;66(9):1550–5.
23. Schulz BS, Wolf G, Hartmann K. Bacteriological and antibiotic sensitivity test results in 271 cats with respiratory tract infections. Vet Rec 2006;158(8):269–70.
24. Sykes JE, Malik R. Cryptococcosis. In: Green CE, editor. Infectious diseases of the dog and cat. 4th edition. St Louis (MO): Elsevier Saunders; 2012. p. 621–34.
25. Reed N, Gunn-Moore D. Nasopharyngeal disease in cats: 1. Diagnostic investigation. J Feline Med Surg 2012;14(5):306–15.
26. Farrow CS, Green R, Shively M. The head. In: Farrow CS, editor. Radiology of the cat. St Louis (MO): Mosby; 1994. p. 1–29.
27. O'Brien RT, Evans SM, Wortman JA, et al. Radiographic findings in cats with intranasal neoplasia or chronic rhinitis: 29 cases (1982–1988). J Am Vet Med Assoc 1996;208(3):385–9.
28. Thrall DE, Robertson ID, McLeod DA, et al. A comparison of radiographic and computed tomographic findings in 31 dogs with malignant nasal cavity tumors. Vet Radiol 1989;30(2):59–65.
29. Park RD, Beck ER, LeCouteur RA. Comparison of computed tomography and radiography for detecting changes induced by malignant nasal neoplasia in dogs. J Am Vet Med Assoc 1992;201(11):1720–4.
30. Codner EC, Lurus AG, Miller JB, et al. Comparison of computed tomography with radiography as a non-invasive diagnostic technique for chronic nasal disease in dogs. J Am Vet Med Assoc 1993;202(7):1106–10.
31. Losonsky JM, Abbott LC, Kuriashkin IV. Computed tomography of the normal feline nasal cavity and paranasal sinuses. Vet Radiol Ultrasound 1997;38(4):251–8.
32. Schoenborn WC, Wisner ER, Kass PP, et al. Retrospective assessment of computed tomographic imaging of feline sinonasal disease in 62 cats. Vet Radiol Ultrasound 2003;44(2):185–95.
33. Tromblee TC, Jones JC, Etue AE, et al. Association between clinical characteristics, computed tomography characteristics, and histologic diagnosis for cats with sinonasal disease. Vet Radiol Ultrasound 2006;47(3):241–8.
34. Johnson LR, Kass PH. Effect of sample collection methodology on nasal culture results in cats. J Feline Med Surg 2009;11(8):645–9.
35. Tomsa K, Glaus TM, Zimmer C, et al. Fungal rhinitis and sinusitis in three cats. J Am Vet Med Assoc 2003;222(10):1380–4.
36. Caniatti M, Roccabianca P, Ghisleni G, et al. Evaluation of brush cytology in the diagnosis of chronic intranasal disease in cats. J Small Anim Pract 1998;39(2):73–7.
37. Elie M, Sabo M. Basics in canine and feline rhinoscopy. Clin Tech Small Anim Pract 2006;21(2):60–3.
38. Johnson LR, Clarke HE, Bannasch MJ, et al. Correlation of rhinoscopic signs of inflammation with histologic findings in nasal biopsy specimens of cats with or without upper respiratory tract disease. J Am Vet Med Assoc 2004;225(3):395–400.
39. Scherk M. Snots and snuffles. Rational approach to chronic feline upper respiratory syndromes. J Feline Med Surg 2010;12(7):548–57.

40. Kuehn N. Chronic rhinitis in cats. Clin Tech Small Anim Pract 2006;21(2): 69–75.
41. Venema CM, Williams KJ, Gershwin LJ, et al. Histopathologic and morphometric evaluation of the nasal and pulmonary airways of cats with experimentally induced asthma. Int Arch Allergy Immunol 2013;160(4):365–76.
42. Sturgess CP, Gruffydd-Jones TJ, Harbour DA, et al. Controlled study of the efficacy of clavulanic acid-potentiated amoxycillin in the treatment of *Chlamydia psittaci* in cats. Vet Rec 2001;149(3):73–6.
43. Owen WM, Sturgess CP, Harbour DA, et al. Efficacy of azithromycin for the treatment of feline chlamydophilosis. J Feline Med Surg 2003;5(6):305–11.
44. Sparkes AH, Caney SM, Sturgess CP, et al. The clinical efficacy of topical and systemic therapy for the treatment of feline ocular chlamydiosis. J Feline Med Surg 1999;1(1):31–5.
45. Hartmann AD, Helps CR, Lapin MR, et al. Efficacy of pradofloxacin in cats with feline upper respiratory tract disease due to *Chlamydophila felis* or *Mycoplasma infections*. J Vet Intern Med 2008;22(1):44–52.
46. Spindel ME, Veir JK, Radecki S, et al. Evaluation of pradofloxacin for the treatment of feline rhinitis. J Feline Med Surg 2008;10(5):472–9.
47. Ruch-Gallie RA, Veir JK, Spindel ME, et al. Efficacy of amoxicillin and azithromycin for the empirical treatment of shelter cats with suspected bacterial upper respiratory infections. J Feline Med Surg 2008;10(6):542–50.
48. Koenig A. Gram-negative bacterial infections. In: Greene CE, editor. Infectious diseases of the dog and cat. 4th edition. St Louis (MO): Elsevier Saunders; 2012. p. 349–59.
49. Court MH, Dodman NH, Seeler DC. Inhalation therapy. Oxygen administration, humidification and aerosol therapy. Vet Clin North Am Small Anim Pract 1985; 15(5):1041–59.
50. Portel L, Turion de Lara JM, Vernejoux JM, et al. Osmolarity of solutions used in nebulisation. Rev Mal Respir 1998;15(2):191–5 [in French].
51. Plumb DC. Plumb's veterinary drug handbook. 6th edition. Ames (IA): Blackwell Publishing Professional; 2008.
52. Ramsey I. BSAVA small animal formulary. 7th edition. Quedgley (England): BSAVA; 2011.
53. Sturgess K. Chronic nasal discharge and sneezing in cats. In Practice 2013;35: 67–74.
54. Hartmann K. Antiviral and immunomodulatory chemotherapy. In: Greene CE, editor. Infectious diseases of the dog and cat. 4th edition. St Louis (MO): Elsevier Saunders; 2012. p. 10–24.
55. Maggs DJ. Antiviral therapy for feline herpesvirus infections. Vet Clin North Am Small Anim Pract 2010;40(6):1055–62.
56. Malik R, Lessels NS, Webb S, et al. Treatment of feline herpesvirus-1 associated disease in cats with famciclovir and related drugs. J Feline Med Surg 2009; 11(1):40–8.
57. Thomasy SM, Lim CC, Reiley CM, et al. Evaluation of famciclovir in cats experimentally infected with feline herpesvirus-1. Am J Vet Res 2011;72(1):85–95.
58. Stiles J, Townsend WM, Rogers QR, et al. Effect of oral administration of L-lysine on conjunctivitis caused by feline herpesvirus in cats. Am J Vet Res 2002;63(1): 99–103.
59. Maggs DJ, Nasisse MP, Kass PH. Efficacy of oral supplementation with L-lysine in cats latently infected with feline herpesvirus. Am J Vet Res 2003; 64(1):37–42.

60. Maggs DJ, Sykes JE, Clarke HE, et al. Effects of dietary lysine supplementation in cats with enzootic upper respiratory disease. J Feline Med Surg 2007;9: 97–108.
61. Rees TM, Lubinski JL. Oral supplementation with L-lysine did not prevent upper respiratory infection in a shelter population of cats. J Feline Med Surg 2008; 10(5):510–3.
62. Drazenovich TL, Fascetti AJ, Westermeyer HD, et al. Effects of dietary lysine supplementation on upper respiratory and ocular disease and detection of infectious organisms in cats within an animal shelter. Am J Vet Res 2009;70(11): 1391–400.
63. Johnson LR, De Cock HE, Sykes JE, et al. Cytokine gene transcription in feline nasal tissue with histologic evidence of inflammation. Am J Vet Res 2005;66(6): 996–1001.
64. Parnes SM. The role of leukotriene inhibitors in patients with paranasal sinus disease. Curr Opin Otolaryngol Head Neck Surg 2003;11(3):184–91.
65. Holmberg DL, Fries C, Cockshutt J, et al. Ventral rhinotomy in the dog and cat. Vet Surg 1989;18(6):446–9.
66. Norsworthy GD. Surgical treatment of chronic nasal discharge in 17 cats. Vet Med 1993;88(6):526–37.
67. Mitten RW. Nasopharyngeal stenosis in four cats. J Small Anim Pract 1988; 29(6):341–5.
68. Mitten R. Acquired nasopharyngeal stenosis in cats. In: Kirk RW, Bonagura JD, editors. Current veterinary therapy X. Philadelphia: WB Saunders; 1992. p. 801–3.
69. Hecht S, Adams WH. MRI of brain disease in veterinary patients. Part 2: acquired brain disorders. Vet Clin North Am Small Anim Pract 2010;40(1):39–63.

Feline Aspergillosis

Vanessa R. Barrs, BVSc(hons), MVetClinStud, FANZCVSc(Feline Medicine), GradCertEd (Higher Ed)*,
Jessica J. Talbot, BSc(vet)(hons)

KEYWORDS

- Aspergillosis • Sinonasal aspergillosis • Sino-orbital aspergillosis • *Aspergillus felis*
- Fungal rhinosinusitis • Antifungals

KEY POINTS

- There are two forms of upper respiratory tract aspergillosis (URTA): sinonasal aspergillosis (SNA) and sino-orbital aspergillosis (SOA). Both infections start in the nasal cavity, and SOA is the most common form (65% of cases).
- Brachycephalic breeds of cats, especially Persian and Himalayan, are predisposed to URTA.
- Feline SNA can be invasive or noninvasive. Noninvasive disease resembles SNA in dogs. The most common causes of SNA are *Aspergillus fumigatus* and *Aspergillus niger*.
- The most common cause of SOA is a recently described novel species, *A felis*, which is an *A fumigatus*-like fungus. Molecular identification is required to differentiate *A felis* from *A fumigatus*.
- The prognosis for SNA is favorable with topical antifungal therapy alone, or combined with systemic antifungals.
- Disseminated and non-URT focal forms of invasive aspergillosis are uncommon in cats, with little known about the etiologic agents. Young to middle-aged cats are affected. Concurrent immunosuppressive diseases have been identified in some cats.

INTRODUCTION

Aspergillosis is a mycosis of a diverse range of human and animal hosts including mammals and birds. Among the most common molds on earth, *Aspergillus* spp. are filamentous ascomycetes distributed primarily in soil and decaying vegetation that have an important role in recycling environmental carbon and nitrogen.[1] The genus is named after "aspergillum," a brush or implement with a perforated head used by Roman Catholic priests for sprinkling holy water, which resembles the fungi's spore-bearing conidial heads.[2]

Faculty of Veterinary Science, University Veterinary Teaching Hospital Sydney, The University of Sydney, Evelyn Williams Building, B10, Sydney, New South Wales 2006, Australia
* Corresponding author.
E-mail address: vanessa.barrs@sydney.edu.au

Vet Clin Small Anim 44 (2014) 51–73
http://dx.doi.org/10.1016/j.cvsm.2013.08.001   vetsmall.theclinics.com

Feline upper respiratory tract aspergillosis (URTA) was first described in the early 1980s.[3] Of the more than 55 cases now reported, over two-thirds were described in the last 5 years.[3–16] Other forms of aspergillosis in cats including disseminated[5,17–21] and focal (non-URT) invasive infections[17,19,20,22–32] are reported less commonly and little is known about the etiologic agents.

CLASSIFICATION SCHEMES

Aspergillosis can be classified by body system involvement, duration of infection, pathology, and pathogenesis. Disease is defined as invasive if there is hyphal invasion into tissues.[33] The respiratory tract is the most common site of disease in humans and animals reflecting the primary inhalational route of infection.

Invasive aspergillosis (IA) in humans occurs predominantly in the sinopulmonary tract of immunocompromised individuals associated with inhalation of *Aspergillus* spp conidia, and invasive pulmonary aspergillosis accounts for more than 90% of IA cases.[34] URTA occurs less commonly and is classified as invasive or noninvasive fungal rhinosinusitis. The classification of sinopulmonary forms of aspergillosis in humans is summarized in **Table 1**.[35–38]

By contrast, URTA is the most common form of aspergillosis reported in mostly immunocompetent cats and dogs.[11,39] URTA can be further subdivided into sinonasal aspergillosis (SNA) and sino-orbital aspergillosis (SOA). In dogs SNA accounts for more than 99% of cases and is noninvasive, whereas in cats SOA is the most common form and is invasive (65% of cases).[3–5,7,8,11,14,16,40–45]

Disseminated IA typically occurs in immunocompromised hosts and is defined as active infection in two or more noncontiguous sites or the hematogenous spread of disease.[35] There are few reports of disseminated IA in cats and most cases had pulmonary involvement.[17–21] Focal (non-URT) invasive infections have also been reported in cats involving lung,[17,19,20,22–25,28] gastrointestinal tract,[20,30–32,46] or urinary bladder.[26,27]

ETIOLOGY

Several hundred species have been ascribed to the genus *Aspergillus*, which includes four major subgenera; *Circumdati*, *Nidulantes*, *Fumigati*, and *Aspergillus*. Each subgenus comprises from two to six sections.[47] The most common isolates to cause URTA in cats and dogs are from the subgenus *Fumigati* section *Fumigati*, also known as the *A fumigatus* complex.[11,48–52] In contrast to dogs, in which *A fumigatus* is the single most common agent of SNA,[53] a more diverse range of *Aspergillus* species has been identified from cases of feline URTA (**Table 2**).[11,12,15,42]

Based on current evidence, *A fumigatus* (section *Fumigati*) and *A niger* (section *Nigri*) are the most common agents of SNA,[9,11,42] whereas a recently discovered species, *A felis* (section *Fumigati*), is the most common cause of SOA followed by *A udagawae* (section *Fumigati*) (see **Table 2**).[12,15,16] Section *Nigri* isolates, known as the black aspergilli, are phenotypically distinct from section *Fumigati* (**Fig. 1**).[54]

Recent Advances in Identification of Fungal Pathogens in URTA

The ability to accurately identify fungal species that cause aspergillosis has increased with the widespread availability of molecular techniques including polymerase chain reaction (PCR) and sequencing.[55] Members of the *A fumigatus* complex cannot be reliably identified on the basis of phenotypic features alone. *A fumigatus*–like or "cryptic" species have similar morphology and other phenotypic features to *A fumigatus*.[51] Misidentification of cryptic species causing feline URTA including

A felis, *A udagawae*, and *A lentulus* is likely when only morphologic typing methods are used.[11,12,51]

In four cases of SOA where *A fumigatus* was reported as the etiologic agent, isolates were identified by phenotypic features alone.[10,43–45] For three of the isolates where antifungal susceptibility to amphotericin B (AMB) was tested, minimum inhibitory concentrations of AMB were high, increasing the likelihood that these isolates were cryptic species.[10,43,44] Compared with *A fumigatus*, the minimum inhibitory concentrations of AMB for cryptic species, such as *A lentulus* and *A udagawae*, are high.[51,56] To date, of 35 cases of feline URTA in which the species identity of isolates was confirmed using PCR and sequencing of the internal transcribed spacer (ITS) and partial β-tubulin genes, *A fumigatus* has only been identified in cases of SNA (see **Table 2**) (Barrs and Talbot, unpublished data, 2013).[11,12,15,16]

Disseminated and Focal IA

The *Aspergillus* spp that cause disseminated IA and focal IA in cats remain largely unknown because most cases were diagnosed at postmortem only from histologic findings.[17–21] *A fumigatus* was identified from fungal culture morphology only in two cats with mycotic pneumonia,[25,28] one cat with mycotic cystitis,[26] and one cat with disseminated IA.[18] *A nidulans* was identified from fungal culture morphology only in one cat with mycotic cystitis.[27] Molecular confirmation of isolate identity was not performed in any case.

Current Fungal Taxonomy: What's in a Name?

The *A fumigatus* complex contains asexual members (anamorphs), many of which also have sexual forms (teleomorphs). The anamorph is typically mold-like and bears mitotic spores (conidia). The teleomorph is characterized by the production of meiotic spores (ascospores) that develop within sacs (asci) inside enclosed fruiting bodies (cleistothecia).[55]

Controversy has surrounded the fungal taxonomy of the *A fumigatus* complex because of the system of dual nomenclature used to describe anamorphic and teleomorphic phases of the same fungus. Traditionally the anamorphic phase was assigned to the genus *Aspergillus*, whereas the teleomorph of the same organism was assigned to the genus *Neosartorya*. The teleomorphic name received taxonomic precedence, such that species with known sexual stages were referred to by their teleomorph names.[57] Although this system of dual nomenclature provided a practical solution for distinguishing organisms that produce ascospores, confusion arose for such organisms as *A fumigatus*, where the teleomorph (*Neosartorya fumigata*) was only recently discovered and the taxon continued to be referred to by its anamorph name.[58]

In reforms to the *International Code of Nomenclature for Algae, Fungi and Plants* a "one-fungus, one-name" principle was adopted in July 2011.[59] In accordance with the Amsterdam declaration on fungal nomenclature, *Neosartorya* is now included in genus *Aspergillus* and teleomorphs are referred to by an informal cross-reference name (eg, *A fumigatus* [neosartorya-morph]).[60]

EPIDEMIOLOGY

Feline URTA occurs worldwide, with cases reported in Australia,[3,11–13,40] the United States,[7–10,41,42,45] Europe,[4,8,14,43] and Japan.[15,16] No age or gender predilection is apparent. The median age at diagnosis is 6.5 years (range, 16 mo to 13 years).[3–5,7,8,11,14,16,40–45]

Table 1
Classification of respiratory aspergillosis in humans

Anatomic Location	Invasive/Noninvasive	Immune Status	Pathology
Lower respiratory tract	IPA (angioinvasive)	Immunocompromised • Prolonged severe neutropenia	Vascular invasion by fungal elements
	IPA (nonangioinvasive)	Immunocompromised nonneutropenic: • HIV/AIDS • Corticosteroids • Hematopoietic stem cell transplant recipients • Heritable immunologic defect (chronic granulomatous disease)	No evidence of vascular invasion Pyogranulomatous inflammatory infiltrate
	Chronic IPA (nonangioinvasive): • Chronic necrotizing PA • Chronic cavitary PA • Chronic fibrosing PA	Immunocompromised: • Structural lung disease (eg, neoplasia, asthma, emphysema, infection) • Corticosteroids • HIV/AIDS • Diabetes • Alcohol abuse	Hyphae mostly contained within cavity with only occasional direct tissue invasion (chronic necrotizing PA)
	Invasive bronchial aspergillosis	Immunocompromised	Hyphal invasion of large airways
	Aspergilloma • Noninvasive	Immunocompetent	Single cavity with fungal ball No hyphal invasion of parenchyma

Upper respiratory tract	Acute invasive FRS (angioinvasive)	Immunocompromised: • Neutropenia • Allogenic stem cell transplant recipients	Hyphal invasion of sinuses and contiguous structures (eg, orbit); coagulative necrosis, sparse inflammatory infiltrate, angioinvasion
	Chronic invasive FRS (angioinvasive)	Immunocompromised: • Diabetes • Corticosteroids • HIV/AIDS	Hyphal invasion of sinuses and contiguous structures (eg, orbit); infiltrative mass, mixed inflammatory response, angioinvasion
	Granulomatous FRS • Invasive	Immunocompetent: • Location-dependent disease (Sudan, Middle-East, Indian subcontinent)	Hyphal invasion of sinuses and contiguous structures (eg, orbit); highly cellular granulomatous inflammatory response, no angioinvasion; similar to feline sino-orbital aspergillosis
	Sinus aspergilloma (fungal ball) • Noninvasive	Immunocompetent: • Structural sinus disease (eg, dental root filling material)	Fungal mass within sinus; chronic nongranulomatous inflammatory response to fungal mass
	Allergic FRS • Noninvasive	Immunocompetent	An allergic/hypersensitivity response to the presence of extramucosal fungi within the sinus
	Chronic erosive noninvasive FRS	Immunocompetent	Similar to canine sinonasal aspergillosis; marked inflammatory response and sinonasal bony lysis

Abbreviations: FRS, fungal rhinosinusitis; IPA, invasive pulmonary aspergillosis; PA, pulmonary aspergillosis.

Table 2
Etiologic agents in genus *Aspergillus* of SNA and SOA in cats

Number of Cases		Identification (Phenotypic[P]/Molecular[M])		
SNA	SOA	Subgenus	Section	Species
7	0	Fumigati	Fumigati	A fumigatus[M]
1	0	Fumigati	Fumigati	A lentulus[M]
1	1	Fumigati	Fumigati	N pseudofischeri (A thermomutatus)[M]
1	18	Fumigati	Fumigati	A felis[M]
0	4	Fumigati	Fumigati	A udagawae[M]
0	1	Fumigati	Fumigati	A virdinutans[M]
3	0	Circumdati	Nigri	A niger[P (n=2), M (n=1)]

Molecular identification is based on polymerase chain reaction and sequencing of the internal transcribed spacer and β-tubulin regions.
Abbreviations: SNA, sinonasal aspergillosis; SOA, sino-orbital aspergillosis.
Data from Refs.[9,11,12,15,16,42]; and Barrs & Talbot unpublished data, 2013.

Of cases where serologic testing for feline immunodeficiency virus and feline leukemia virus was performed, only one cat tested positive for feline leukemia virus.[4] Diabetes mellitus, a recognized risk factor for aspergillosis in humans (see **Table 1**), was present in two cats diagnosed with URTA.[40,42] As has been reported in canine SNA,[39,61,62] feline URTA occurs occasionally in association with facial trauma, nasal neoplasia, and nasal foreign bodies (Barrs, unpublished data, 2013).

In contrast to canine SNA where dolicocephalic and mesaticephalic breeds are overrepresented,[39] pure-bred brachycephalic cats, predominantly of Persian or Himalayan breed, account for more than a third of all feline URTA cases.[3–5,7,8,11,14,16,40–45]

No gender or breed predisposition has been recorded for disseminated and focal IA in cats. Affected cats are usually young to middle-aged. Evidence of systemic immunocompromise in some cases included feline panleukopenia virus infection, feline leukemia virus infection, feline infectious peritonitis, or prolonged corticosteroid therapy.[17–21,30–32,46]

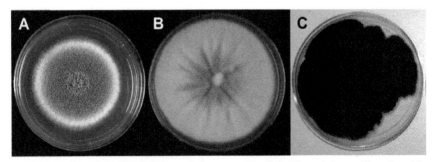

Fig. 1. Isolates of *Aspergillus fumigatus* (*A*), *Aspergillus felis* (*B*), and *Aspergillus niger* (*C*) on malt extract agar, from cats with URT aspergillosis. The black aspergilli (Section *Nigri*; [*C*]) are phenotypically distinct from Section *Fumigati* (*A*, *B*). Species within Section *Fumigati* cannot be reliably identified from phenotypic features. Some, like *A felis* (*B*), are generally slow to sporulate.

PATHOGENESIS

The ability of fungi to cause disease depends on a complex interplay between the pathogen (virulence factors) and the host (innate and adaptive immune responses). In humans, host factors that predispose individuals to IA include disorders of innate immunity, such as reduced mucociliary clearance (eg, cystic fibrosis); decreased numbers of phagocytic cells (ie, neutropenia); and phagocytic cell dysfunction (eg, chronic granulomatous disease, in which there is impaired production of oxidative intermediates).[63]

After inhalation, *Aspergillus* conidia that escape mucociliary clearance are mostly phagocytosed by macrophages and dendritic cells.[34] Phagocytic host cells express pattern recognition receptors (PRRs) that recognize specific fungal epitopes known as pathogen-associated molecular patterns (PAMPs) and damaged host cell components known as damage-associated molecular patterns (DAMPs). The major PAMPs of filamentous fungi are cell-wall components including β-glucans, chitin, and mannans, whereas DAMPs include nucleic acids and alarmins. The major PRRs of host cells, as characterized in humans, include C-type lectin receptors; toll-like receptors (TLRs); nucleotide oligomerization domain-like receptors (NOD-like receptors or NLRs); and galectin family proteins.[63,64]

Is URTA Associated with a Disorder of Innate Immunity?

To date no studies have been performed to investigate innate or immune responses in cats with URTA. Several single nucleotide polymorphisms in PRRs that increase susceptibility to IA have been described in humans including single nucleotide polymorphisms in TLRs 1, 3, 4, and 6, and in the C-type lectin receptors Dectin-1 and DC-SIGN.[64,65] Whether similar genetic mutations could be associated with increased susceptibility to URTA in Persian/Himalayan cats has not been investigated. By contrast, several studies have evaluated the immune response to SNA in dogs.[66–69] It is characterized by a dominant T-helper cell 1 (Th1) response with upregulation of interleukin-10. A dominant Th1 response correlates with protective antifungal immunity and is thought to be important in preventing invasive disease.[39] Upregulation of interleukin-10 is important in limiting the extent of local tissue destruction[70] but paradoxically could also be the reason why affected dogs are unable to clear infection spontaneously. The inflammatory process in fungal infection is beneficial in containing the infection but an uncontrolled inflammatory response is detrimental and might inhibit disease eradication.[64]

To explore the hypothesis that a dysfunction in innate immunity could be an etiologic factor in the development of canine SNA, the expression of messenger RNA (mRNA) encoding TLRs 1 to 10 and NLRs 1 and 2 was quantified in nasal mucosal biopsies from dogs with SNA and control dogs using quantitative real-time PCR.[68] In dogs with SNA there was significantly higher expression of all PRRs except for TLR3, TLR5, and NLR1 compared with normal dogs. The significance of these findings is unknown because little is known about the function of PRRs in canine nasal immunity in health and disease.

Is URTA Associated with Impaired Mucociliary Clearance?

The increased risk of URTA observed in brachycephalic cats could reflect reduced mucociliary clearance from abnormal sinonasal cavity conformation. Decreased sinus aeration and drainage of respiratory secretions secondary to infection, polyps, and allergic rhinosinusitis is a risk factor for invasive fungal rhinosinusitis in humans.[71] Mucosal edema and impaired drainage of URT secretions caused by turbulent airflow and abnormal facial conformation has been proposed as a risk factor for fungal colonization in brachycephalic cats.[8] However, because brachycephalic dogs are underrepresented for SNA, additional risk factors, such as previous viral URT infection or recurrent antimicrobial therapy, could also be involved.[4,8,11]

Fungal Virulence Factors

An important virulence factor of *Aspergillus* spp is their thermotolerant nature that enables survival in mammals.[72] Toxic secondary metabolites are associated with host immunosuppression or evasion of the immune system.[73] Gliotoxin, a mycelial-derived product, prevents phagocytosis by macrophages, reduces T-cell proliferation and activation, and induces macrophage apoptosis.[73–75] Other putative fungal virulence factors include the ability to adhere to host tissue by conidia and laminin-binding components, factors interfering with fungal cell opsonization, and the production of proteases capable of macromolecule degradation to provide fungal nutrients.[73] Species-specific fungal virulence factors could be involved in the development of invasive URTA because different fungal species are implicated in SNA and SOA in cats.[12]

Progression from SNA to SOA

SOA results from extension of a primary sinonasal infection to involve paranasal structures including, but not limited to the orbit. The evidence for this includes:

- Documented progression of disease from SNA to SOA.[7]
- History of nasal signs preceding development of an orbital fungal granuloma.[3,7,11,16,45]
- Detection of concurrent sinonasal cavity involvement on imaging, at surgery, or at necropsy.[3,6,10,11]
- Detection of a direct communication between the orbit and nasal cavity on computed tomography, surgery, or necropsy in the orbital lamina and less commonly the frontal bone.[11,43,76]
- Isolation of *A felis*, the most common cause of SOA, from a cat with SNA.[12] A large defect in the orbital lamina was present on computed tomography. Infection was arrested with aggressive antifungal therapy and SOA did not develop.[11]

CLINICAL PRESENTATION

Clinical findings in feline SNA (outlined in **Box 1**) are similar to those reported for chronic rhinosinusitis (discussed elsewhere in this issue). Most cats with SOA are presented for clinical signs associated with an invasive retrobulbar fungal granuloma (**Box 2, Fig. 2**).[3,7,10,11,14–16,43–45] In most cats exophthalmos is unilateral, but in severe, chronic infections, bilateral exophthalmos can occur.[3,11,43] Nasal signs are absent in 40% of SOA cases at presentation; however, the medical history usually reveals sneezing or nasal discharge in the preceding 6 months. Pain on opening the mouth and neurologic signs are uncommon at initial presentation. However, cats with advanced disease are often euthanized because of the development of neurologic signs, which can include seizures, nystagmus, circling, facial muscle fasciculation, hyperesthesia, and blindness.[11,44,45]

DIFFERENTIAL DIAGNOSES

Differential diagnoses for cats presenting with chronic nasal signs are listed in **Box 3** and for cats presenting with exophthalmos are listed in **Box 4**. Brachycephalic

---

Box 1
Clinical signs in sinonasal aspergillosis

Common signs

- Sneezing
- Stertor
- Unilateral or bilateral serous to mucopurulent nasal discharge
- Ipsilateral mild mandibular lymphadenopathy

Less common signs

- Epistaxis (30% of cases)
- Fever
- Discharging sinus or soft tissue mass involving the nasal bone or frontal sinus

---

conformation should increase suspicion for aspergillosis, although these cats are also overrepresented for viral URT infections. Where epistaxis is present neoplasia, mycotic rhinitis, or severe chronic rhinosinusitis are more likely, along with systemic hypertension. Inability to retropulse the globe and measurement of intraocular pressure enables differentiation of exophthalmos from buphthalmos (abnormal enlargement of the globe).[45] Other infectious or neoplastic processes extending from the nasal cavity to the orbit can have a similar presentation to SOA, including cryptococcosis, nasal lymphoma, and nasal carcinoma.

Box 2
Clinical signs in sino-orbital aspergillosis

Common signs

- Nasal signs (clinical or historical finding within the previous 6 months)
- Unilateral exophthalmos with dorsolateral deviation of the globe
- Ipsilateral conjunctival hyperemia
- Ipsilateral prolapse of the nictitating membrane
- Ipsilateral exposure keratitis
- Oral mass or ulcer in the ipsilateral pterygopalatine fossa
- Paranasal soft tissue swelling
- Nasal signs
- Mild mandibular lymphadenopathy

Less common signs

- Fever
- Bilateral exophthalmos
- Ulceration of the hard palate
- Neurologic signs
- Discharging sinus (facial)

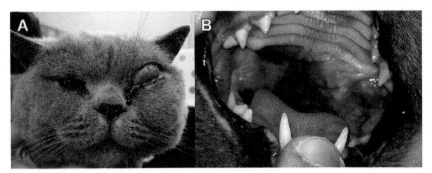

Fig. 2. British Shorthair cat with sino-orbital aspergillosis. Infection was caused by *Aspergillus felis*. Note the left-sided third eyelid prolapse, hyperemia, and edema, and the paranasal soft tissue swelling (*A*), and the pterygopalatine fossa mass (*B*), caused by an invasive retrobulbar fungal granuloma.

DIAGNOSIS

Diagnosis of feline URTA requires various combinations of serology, advanced imaging, rhinosinuscopy, cytology, histology, fungal culture, and molecular identification. Definitive diagnosis is based on identification of fungal hyphae on cytologic or histologic examination of tissue biopsies or sinonasal fungal plaques. Similar to canine SNA, diagnosis can also be made by visualization of sinonasal fungal plaques on endoscopy.[4,42] However, given the more diverse range of fungal pathogens that can cause feline URTA, definitive identification of fungal pathogens should always be attempted.

Hematology and Biochemistry

Hematology is unremarkable or there is evidence of a stress or inflammatory leukogram. Peripheral eosinophilia is uncommon (10% of cases).[7,8,10,11,16,42–45] Mild to severe hyperglobulinemia is the most common abnormality on serum biochemistry. This was reported in 9 of 16 cats with SOA and one cat with SNA caused by *A felis* infection.[7,10,11,45] This finding suggests that in cats with confirmed URTA the presence of hyperglobulinemia is a marker for invasive disease. However, prospective studies are required to investigate this.

Box 3
Differential diagnoses of nasal signs

Neoplasia (lymphoma, carcinoma, other)

Inflammatory (chronic rhinosinusitis, nasal/nasopharyngeal polyp, nasopharyngeal stenosis)

Infectious

  Viral (Feline Herpesvirus-1, Feline Calicivirus)

  Mycotic rhinitis (cryptococcosis, aspergillosis, sporotrichosis, phaeohyphomycoses, other)

  Bacterial (*Bordetella*, *Mycoplasma*, *Chlamydophila felis*, *Actinomycetes*)

Foreign body

Congenital (choanal atresia, palatine defects)

Dental disease (oronasal fistula)

Box 4
Differential diagnoses of orbital mass lesions

Neoplasia

  Lymphoma

  Adenocarcinoma/undifferentiated carcinoma

  Squamous cell carcinoma

  Fibrosarcoma

  Osteoma/osteosarcoma

  Other

Infectious

  Bacterial abscess/granuloma (odontogenic, penetrating bite wound, hematogenous)

  Mycotic granuloma

    Aspergillosis

    Cryptococcosis

    Penicilliosis

    Phaeohyphomycosis

    Hyalohyphomycosis

  Pythiosis

Inflammatory

  Orbital myofascitis

  Orbital pseudotumor (idiopathic sclerosing inflammation)

  Zygomatic or lacrimal adenitis

Foreign body (eg, grass awn)

Orbital fat prolapse

Serology

Aspergillus antigen detection in URTA

Galactomannan (GM) is a polysaccharide component of the cell wall of *Aspergillus* and other filamentous fungal species that is released into the circulation during hyphal invasion into tissue.[77] A recent study evaluated serum GM measurement for diagnosis of feline URTA.[78] A one-stage, immunoenzymatic sandwich enzyme-linked immunosorbent assay (ELISA) (Platelia, Bio-Rad, Marnes-la-Coquette, France) was used to detect serum GM in four groups of cats: Group 1 cats had confirmed URTA (N = 13; six SNA, seven SOA); Group 2 cats had other URT diseases (N = 15); Group 3 cats were treated with β-lactam antibiotics for non–respiratory tract disease (N = 14); and Group 4 were healthy cats (Group 4a cats ≤1 year of age, N = 28; Group 4b cats >1 year of age, N = 16). Using a cut-off optical density index of 1.5, 3 of 13 cats with URTA (two SOA, one SNA) tested positive for serum GM. The overall sensitivity and specificity of the assay was 23% and 78%, respectively. False-positive results occurred in 29% of cats in Group 3 and 32% of cats in Group 4a. Specificity increased to 90% when Groups 3 and 4a were excluded from the analysis.

    The low sensitivity of detection of serum GM in feline URTA is likely to be associated with systemic immunocompetence of the host. In humans, the sensitivity of the

GM ELISA for detection of IA is more than 90% in neutropenic patients,[79] whereas in nonneutropenic patients the sensitivity is less than 30%.[80,81] In the former, antigen is cleared by neutrophils, which possess mannose-binding receptors, or by complexing with circulating anti-*Aspergillus* antibodies.[82,83] Also, low sensitivity of GM detection in feline SNA could reflect absence of tissue invasion, as is the case in canine SNA where fungal hyphae colonize superficially but do not penetrate the sinonasal epithelium.[84]

The poor specificity of the Platelia GM assay for diagnosis of feline URTA mimics the situation in humans where false-positive results have been identified in pediatric patients, and in patients treated with β-lactam antibiotics that contain small amounts of GM introduced during the manufacturing process.[85,86] Except in the setting of ruling out URTA in cats with respiratory disease, serum GM is not useful as a routine diagnostic test for feline URTA.

Antibody tests

Serum anti-*Aspergillus* antibodies can be detected by numerous methods including counter-immunoelectrophoresis, agar gel immunodiffusion, or ELISA. Results of serologic tests performed in commercial laboratories have been published in case-reports totaling 10 cats with URTA (nine SNA, one SOA), of which five were seropositive.[4,8,9,11,42]

Preliminary results of a prospective study to evaluate the diagnostic sensitivity and specificity of anti-*Aspergillus* antibody detection in feline URTA indicate that antibodies to *A felis* cross-react with the same aspergillin preparation evaluated for diagnosis of canine SNA (Aspergillus Immunodiffusion Antigen, Meridian Bioscience, Cincinnati, Ohio, USA) (Barrs, unpublished data, 2013).

Diagnostic Imaging: Computed Tomography and Magnetic Resonance Imaging

Advanced imaging (computed tomography [CT] or magnetic resonance imaging [MRI]) is recommended for all cases of suspected feline URTA. As for canine SNA, cribriform plate integrity should be assessed before treatment with topical antifungal preparations. Evidence of invasive disease, including paranasal soft tissue infiltration and orbital involvement, may not be apparent on physical examination. Determination of orbital involvement will affect subsequent case management.[11] CT is generally superior to MRI for evaluation of destructive lesions in bony structures contiguous with the sinonasal cavity. In cats with suspected intracranial extension of infection, MRI after intravenous contrast administration is superior to CT for evaluation of intracranial soft tissues.

CT findings in SNA

CT findings in cats with SNA have been reported in a small number of cases and seem to be more variable than in canine SNA.[9,41,42,76] Common findings are listed in **Box 5**. In one study of five cats with SNA, findings that are relatively specific for SNA in dogs, including cavitated-like turbinate lysis, mucosal rim thickening adjacent to the bones of the sinonasal cavity, soft tissue accumulation, and reactive bony-changes, were absent.[41] However, these changes have been observed recently in cats with SNA caused by *A fumigatus* (Barrs, unpublished data, 2013).

A calcified nasal cavity concretion was reported in one case of feline SNA.[8] Calcification of fungal plaques occurs in sinonasal *Aspergillus* spp infections in humans, in approximately 50% of non-IA sinus fungal balls with maxillary sinus involvement.[87] It is caused by deposition of calcium oxalate or phosphate crystals that are thought to be fungal metabolites.

```
┌─────────────────────────────────────────────────────────────────────┐
│ Box 5                                                                 │
│ CT findings in SNA                                                    │
├─────────────────────────────────────────────────────────────────────┤
│                                                                       │
│ • Nasal cavity involvement is usually bilateral                       │
│                                                                       │
│ • Turbinate lysis                                                     │
│                                                                       │
│ • Increased soft tissue attenuation within the nasal cavities         │
│                                                                       │
│ • Fluid or soft tissue accumulation within frontal and sphenoid sinuses│
│                                                                       │
│ Additional CT findings in SOA                                         │
│                                                                       │
│ • Ventromedial orbital mass                                           │
│                                                                       │
│ • Dorsolateral displacement of the globe, which may be indented       │
│                                                                       │
│ • Heterogeneous and peripheral rim post contrast enhancement of orbital mass│
│                                                                       │
│ • Paranasal soft tissue mass effect: pterygopalatine fossa, adjacent maxilla│
│                                                                       │
│ • Lytic lesions in paranasal bones                                    │
│                                                                       │
└─────────────────────────────────────────────────────────────────────┘
```

CT findings in SOA

CT Features of SOA (see **Box 5**) overlap those seen in malignant nasal neoplasia (eg, nasal lymphoma, nasal carcinomas) and other invasive mycoses, such as cryptococcosis (**Fig. 3**).[41] Overlapping features include osteolysis of paranasal bones, moderate to severe turbinate destruction, mass-effect, and extension of disease into the orbit or paranasal soft tissues.[43–45,76,88,89]

Biopsy Procedures

Endoscopic visualization of the sinonasal cavity can be performed using nasopharyngoscopy, rhinoscopy, and sinuscopy. Biopsy specimens are obtained for cytology and/or histology, and culture. Biopsy specimens can be stored frozen for PCR if URTA is suspected but fungal culture is negative. Nasal cavity lavage may yield larger biopsy specimens than can be acquired endoscopically and assists in debridement of mucosal plaques (**Fig. 4**).

Sinuscopy is indicated when CT findings indicate sinus involvement and fungal plaques are not visualized on rhinoscopy. Anatomic landmarks have been defined for sinus trephination in cats.[90] Trephine openings are made slightly to the side of the mid-line on a line that joins the anterior borders of the supraorbital processes.

For cats with SOA, biopsies of retrobulbar masses can be obtained by the oral cavity where there is pterygopalatine invasion.[11] CT-guided biopsies of orbital or other paranasal mass lesions can be performed.[45]

Fungal culture

Fungal pathogens that cause feline URTA can be readily cultured from tissue biopsies or fungal plaques using commercial culture media. In one study 22 of 23 cases of feline URTA were culture positive.[11] Culture of nasal swabs for diagnosis of feline URTA has not been evaluated.

Molecular identification of fungi

In the clinical setting comparative DNA sequence analysis used in conjunction with traditional phenotype-based methods is a practical approach to identification of species within the genus *Aspergillus*.[52] Fungal DNA can be extracted for sequencing directly from fresh or frozen clinical specimens, or from fungal culture material. One

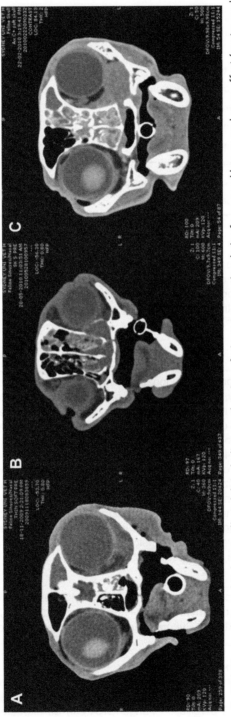

Fig. 3. CT features of sino-orbital aspergillosis (A), including nasal cavity soft tissue attenuation, lysis of paranasal bones, and mass-effect (ventromedial orbital mass), overlap those of other mycoses (eg, cryptococcosis) (B), and neoplasia (eg, lymphoma) (C).

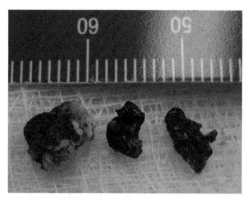

Fig. 4. Plaques of *Aspergillus fumigatus* retrieved from the nasopharynx of a cat after nasal lavage under general anesthesia, with sterile saline.

of the limitations of using formalin-fixed paraffin embedded tissues is that they often only yield short DNA fragments, thus limiting the gene targets for amplification.

The genome of all fungi contains multiple copies of the ribosomal DNA (rDNA) gene complex, consisting of highly variable regions, the ITS regions, which are flanked by highly conserved gene sequences that are suitable targets for primers. Sequence heterogeneity within the ITS regions is useful for the separation of genera and species, and appropriately exploited as a "panfungal" PCR for identification of fungi in clinical specimens.[91,92] The rDNA gene complex includes three genes: (1) the 18s rDNA gene, also known as the small-subunit rDNA gene, which is 1800 base pairs (bp) long; (2) the 5.8S gene (159 bp); and (3) the 28S rDNA, also known as the large-subunit rDNA gene (3396 bp) (**Fig. 5**).[93] Comparative sequence analysis of ITS1-5.8S-ITS2 is an appropriate locus to first identify *Aspergillus* isolates to the level of subgenus/complex.[52] However, because some closely related species show little or no variation in ITS sequences, accurate identification of the fungal species requires additional analyses of one or more partial gene regions.[94]

Histopathology

SNA
Histologic changes in canine SNA are characterized by ulcerated and severely inflamed mucosa, often covered by a plaque of necrotic tissue containing hyphae, and/or luminal exudates containing hyphae.[9,42,84] Fungal hyphae do not penetrate the mucosal epithelium, and the underlying lamina propria is typically heavily infiltrated by a dense sheet of mixed mononuclear inflammatory cells. Histologic changes in noninvasive feline SNA have not been reported systematically but seem similar to canine SNA. Changes include severe inflammatory rhinitis with lymphoplasmacytic

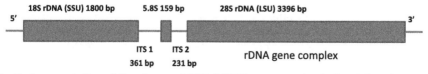

Fig. 5. Representation of the ribosomal DNA (rDNA) gene complex in fungi denoting gene order of small subunit (SSU) and large subunit (LSU) and position of internal transcribed spacer (ITS) regions.

or mixed-cell inflammatory cell infiltrates; necrosis, which can be extensive; and mats of fungal hyphae.[8,9,11,42] Histopathologic detection of tissue invasion by fungal hyphae is important because progression to SOA can occur in invasive infections, and evidence of invasion affects treatment decisions (discussed later).[8]

SOA

Cats with SOA have granulomatous invasive mycotic rhinitis and sinusitis with variable submucosal invasion and bony lysis.[3,11,43] Granulomas are comprised of central necrotic cellular debris within which parallel-walled dichotomously branching, septate fungal hyphae are confined that can be readily identified using special stains (eg, periodic acid–Schiff, Grocott methenamine silver, or Gridley stain).[3,7,10,11,43,45] Surrounding the central area of coagulative necrosis are zones of inflammatory cells and peripheral fibrosis that wall off the hyphae. In some lesions eosinophilic inflammation is prolific, whereas in others neutrophilic inflammation is predominant. Adjacent to these are activated and epithelioid macrophages with vacuolated cytoplasm that form sheets in some places. Peripherally there is a zone of fibroblasts and a cuff of lymphocytes and plasma cells. Inflammatory lesions can efface adjacent skeletal muscle and bone.[11] The globe is resistant to infiltration by fungal hyphae; however, invasion of adjacent structures including the nictitating membrane and eyelid has been observed (Barrs and Day MJ, unpublished data, 2011).[10,44] Mycotic invasion of the optic nerve and optic chiasm in cats that developed blindness has been reported.[11] Development of central nervous system signs in some cases implies fungal invasion of central nervous system tissue; however, brain histology was not performed in the two cats in which seizures were described.[44,45]

TREATMENT AND PROGNOSIS
SNA

The prognosis for feline SNA is favorable, although only small numbers of cases have been treated. Signs resolved in 11 of 14 treated cases in which follow-up information was available.[4,8,9,11,42] Successful treatment regimes included systemic antifungal therapy alone in five cases (itraconazole or posaconazole monotherapy or combined with AMB); systemic triazole therapy (itraconazole or posaconazole) and topical intranasal clotrimazole infusion in two cases; and topical intranasal clotrimazole infusion alone in two cases. As for canine SNA,[95] debridement of fungal lesions in the nasal cavity was an important part of therapy for most cases.[4,8,11,42]

Evidence-based treatment protocols are not available. A suggested therapeutic strategy for treatment of feline SNA, based on previous reports, treatment of canine SNA, and considering whether infection is invasive or noninvasive, is outlined in **Box 6**. Because of the propensity for feline SNA to progress to SOA, where there is any doubt about the presence of invasion, or where *A felis*, a species highly correlated with invasive disease, is identified, concurrent topical and systemic therapy is recommended.

Techniques for intranasal clotrimazole infusion are adapted from procedures used to treat canine SNA and are described in detail elsewhere.[8,39,42] Polyethylene glycol should be used as the vehicle for 1% intranasal clotrimazole infusions, not polypropylene glycol, because the latter can cause severe mucosal edema and ulceration.[96] Response to therapy can be assessed from repeat CT and endoscopy. As for canine SNA, multiple clotrimazole infusions may be required to resolve infection.[11]

SOA

SOA carries a poor prognosis. Optimal treatment protocols for treatment of SOA have not been identified. Based on treatment responses in individual cases[7,10,11,16,45] the

---

Box 6
Therapeutic approach for treatment of feline SNA

- Record the identity of the fungal isolate and its antifungal susceptibility.

- Assess whether infection is invasive or noninvasive based on histopathology and CT findings.

- Determine the integrity of the cribriform plate on CT.

- Debride fungal plaques/lesions from the nasal cavity and frontal sinuses using endoscopic techniques and saline irrigation.

- For noninvasive infections instill an intranasal infusion of 1% clotrimazole in polyethylene glycol (1 hour soak under general anesthesia). Ensure drainage of the infusion from the nasal cavities at the end of the procedure by tilting the head.

- For invasive infections or where *Aspergillus felis* is identified, give additional systemic antifungal therapy (see SOA treatment).

---

recommended therapeutic approach is posaconazole or itraconazole given as mono-therapy or combined with AMB (**Table 3**). Administration of systemic antifungals for 6 months or longer can be necessary in some cases and reinfection or relapse of infection can occur.[11,16] *A felis*, the most common cause of SOA, usually shows in vitro susceptibility to AMB.[12] AMB was used in the successful treatment of one case of SNA and one case of SOA caused by *A felis*, in combination with itraconazole or posaconazole.[11]

Surgical debridement of large granulomas is logical but a clear advantage over medical therapy has not been demonstrated in SOA. Three of six cases that responded to therapy had surgery including orbital exenteration in two cases and debridement of the orbital granuloma in the other.[7,10,45] One of these also had lavage of orbital tissues at surgery with 1% voriconazole.[45] In only one of these cases was resolution of infection confirmed by follow-up CT[10] and one cat was euthanized 4 months after exenteration, with likely progressive disease.[7] In the largest case series of 12 cats with SOA for which treatment outcomes could be assessed, there were 11 treatment failures including five cases treated with combined surgery and antifungal therapy and six with medical therapy alone. One case treated successfully with medical therapy alone relapsed 19 months after treatment was stopped, responded to further medical therapy, and is disease free 5 years later.[11]

Fluconazole is not recommended for treatment of aspergillosis because most *Aspergillus* species are resistant to this drug. Antifungal susceptibility testing should be performed before treatment, because resistance to AMB and some triazole drugs has been identified in isolates from cases of SOA.[10,12,43,44]

Establishing pretreatment renal function and base-line liver enzymes is also important because nephrotoxicity and hepatotoxicity is common with some antifungal drugs (see **Table 3**).

Voriconazole (structurally similar to fluconazole) and posaconazole (structurally similar to itraconazole) are fungicidal triazoles that were developed as more efficacious agents for treatment and prophylaxis of IA in humans and to improve on the absorption, tolerability, and drug interaction profile of itraconazole. Although their pharmacologic characteristics have not been determined in cats, posaconazole is well tolerated after oral administration and liver enzyme elevations are infrequent.[10,11,44] Serious adverse neurologic effects (hindlimb paraplegia and blindness) were reported after voriconazole administration in cats,[11,45,97] and it is not recommended for treatment of feline URTA unless other therapies have failed.

Table 3
Dosages of antifungals used in the treatment of feline upper respiratory tract aspergillosis

Drug/Formulation	Dosage/Route of Administration	Adverse Effects
Itraconazole 100-mg capsules 10 mg/mL oral suspension (Sporanox)	Capsules: 5 mg/kg q 12 h or 10 mg/kg q 24 h PO Administer with food Oral suspension: 1–1.5 mg/kg q 24 h PO	Gastrointestinal: anorexia, vomiting Hepatotoxicity: elevated liver enzyme levels, jaundice. Monitor ALP/ALT monthly. If hepatotoxicity occurs, reduce dosage to 5 mg/kg q 24 h or 10 mg/kg q 48 h PO (capsules)
Posaconazole 40 mg/mL liquid (Noxafil)	5–7.5 mg/kg divided twice daily PO Administer with food	Hepatotoxicity: unlikely to occur at 5 mg/kg divided twice daily PO
Voriconazole 50-mg tablets 40 mg/mL powder for oral suspension (Vfend)	5 mg/kg q 24 h PO	Gastrointestinal: anorexia Neurologic: blindness, ataxia, stupor, hind-limb paraplegia. Consider use only when other therapies have failed
Terbinafine 250-mg tablets (Lamisil)	30 mg/kg q 24 h PO	Gastrointestinal: anorexia, vomiting, diarrhea
Amphotericin B deoxycholate 50-mg vial (Fungizone)	0.5 mg/kg of 5 mg/mL stock solution in 350 mL per cat of 0.45% NaCl + 2.5% dextrose SC two or three times weekly to a cumulative dose of 10–15 mg/kg	Nephrotoxicity: monitor urea/creatinine every 2 wk. Discontinue for 2–3 wk if azotemic
Liposomal amphotericin (AmBisome)	1–1.5 mg/kg IV q 48 h to a cumulative dose of 12–15 mg/kg Give as a 1–2 mg/mL solution in 5% dextrose by IV infusion over 1–2 h	Nephrotoxicity: less nephrotoxic than amphotericin B, but azotemia can occur. Monitor urea/creatinine 1–2 × weekly

Echinocandins, a novel class of semisynthetic amphiphilic lipopetides, inhibit synthesis of the fungal cell wall component 1,3-β-glucan. They are used for treatment of refractory IA in humans.[98] Caspofungin was well tolerated and efficacious in one cat with SOA that failed treatment with AMB and posaconazole.[11] In another case treatment with micafungin was unsuccessful.[15] As with other polypeptides, echinocandins can cause histamine release.

SUMMARY

Feline URTA, the most commonly reported form of aspergillosis in cats, commences as an infection in the nasal cavity. In SNA, infections remain confined to the sinonasal cavity. In SOA, which is an invasive mycosis, infection extends from the nasal cavity to involve paranasal structures, including the orbit. In contrast to canine SNA, feline URTA is caused by a diverse range of *Aspergillus* species, mostly from the *A fumigatus* complex. Phenotypic methods of identification are unreliable, but fungi can be readily identified using PCR and sequencing of the ITS and β-tubulin gene regions. SNA carries a favorable prognosis with treatment, whereas the prognosis for SOA is poor. Optimal treatment regimes for feline URTA have not been identified.

REFERENCES

1. Latge JP. *Aspergillus fumigatus* and aspergillosis. Clin Microbiol Rev 1999; 12(2):310–50.
2. Bennett JW. Aspergillus: a primer for the novice. Med Mycol 2009;47:S5–12.
3. Wilkinson GT, Sutton RH, Grono LR. *Aspergillus* spp infection associated with orbital cellulitis and sinusitis in a cat. J Small Anim Pract 1982;23(3):127–31.
4. Goodall SA, Lane JG, Warnock DW. The diagnosis and treatment of a case of nasal aspergillosis in a cat. J Small Anim Pract 1984;25(10):627–33.
5. Davies C, Troy GC. Deep mycotic infections in cats. J Am Anim Hosp Assoc 1996;32(5):380–91.
6. Halenda RM, Reed AL. Ultrasound computed tomography diagnosis: fungal, sinusitis and retrobulbar myofascitis in a cat. Vet Radiol Ultrasound 1997; 38(3):208–10.
7. Hamilton HL, Whitley RD, McLaughlin SA. Exophthalmos secondary to aspergillosis in a cat. J Am Anim Hosp Assoc 2000;36(4):343–7.
8. Tomsa K, Glaus TA, Zimmer C, et al. Fungal rhinitis and sinusitis in three cats. J Am Vet Med Assoc 2003;222(10):1380–4.
9. Whitney BL, Broussard J, Stefanacci JD. Four cats with fungal rhinitis. J Feline Med Surg 2005;7(1):53–8.
10. McLellan GJ, Aquino SM, Mason DR, et al. Use of posaconazole in the management of invasive orbital aspergillosis in a cat. J Am Anim Hosp Assoc 2006; 42(4):302–7.
11. Barrs VR, Halliday C, Martin P, et al. Sinonasal and sino-orbital aspergillosis in 23 cats: aetiology, clinicopathological features and treatment outcomes. Vet J 2012;191(1):58–64.
12. Barrs VR, van Doorn T, Houbraken J, et al. *Aspergillus felis* sp. nov., an emerging agent of invasive aspergillosis in humans, cats and dogs. PLoS One 2013;8(6):e64871.
13. Katz ME, Dougall AM, Weeks K, et al. Multiple genetically distinct groups revealed among clinical isolates identified as atypical *Aspergillus fumigatus*. J Clin Microbiol 2005;43(2):551–5.
14. Declercq J, Declercq L, Fincioen S. Unilateral sino-orbital and subcutaneous aspergillosis in a cat. Vlaams Diergeneeskd Tijdschr 2012;81(6):357–62.
15. Kano R, Itamoto K, Okuda M, et al. Isolation of *Aspergillus udagawae* from a fatal case of feline orbital aspergillosis. Mycoses 2008;51(4):360–1.
16. Kano R, Shibahashi A, Fujino Y, et al. Two cases of feline orbital aspergillosis due to *A. udagawae* and *A. virdinutans*. J Vet Med Sci 2013;75:7–10.
17. Fox JG, Murphy JC, Shalev M. Systemic fungal infections in cats. J Am Vet Med Assoc 1978;173(9):1191–5.
18. Vogler GA, Wagner JE. What's your diagnosis. Lab Anim 1975;5:14.
19. Köhler H, Kuttin E, Kaplan W, et al. Occurence of systemic mycoses in animals in Austria. Zentralbl Veterinarmed B 1978;25(10):785–99.
20. Ossent P. Systemic aspergillosis and mucormycosis in 23 cats. Vet Rec 1987; 120(14):330–3.
21. Burk RL, Joseph R, Baer K. Systemic aspergillosis in a cat. Vet Radiol Ultrasound 1990;31(1):26–8.

22. Sautter JH, Steele DS, Henry JF. Symposium on granulomatous diseases II. J Am Vet Med Assoc 1955;127:518.
23. Pakes SP, New AE, Benbrook SC. Pulmonary aspergillosis in a cat. J Am Vet Med Assoc 1967;151(7):950-3.
24. McCausland IP. Systemic mycoses of two cats. N Z Vet J 1972;20(1-2):10-2.
25. Hazell KL, Swift IM, Sullivan N. Successful treatment of pulmonary aspergillosis in a cat. Aust Vet J 2011;89(3):101-4.
26. Kirkpatrick RM. Mycotic cystitis in a male cat. Vet Med Small Anim Clin 1982;77: 1365-71.
27. Adamama-Moraitou KK, Paitaki CG, Rallis TS, et al. Aspergillus species cystitis in a cat. J Feline Med Surg 2001;3:31-4.
28. Degi J, Radbea G, Balaban S, et al. Aspergillus pneumonia in a Burmese cat: case study. Lucrari Stiintifice - Universitatea de Stiinte Agricole a Banatului Timisoara, Medicina Veterinara 2011;44(2):278-81.
29. Schiefer B. Dtsch Tierarztl Wochenschr 1965;72:73.
30. Weiland F. Intestinal mycosis in a cat. Dtsch Tierarztl Wochenschr 1970;77(10): 232-3.
31. Bolton GR, Brown TT. Mycotic colitis in a cat. Vet Med Small Anim Clin 1972; 67(9):978-81.
32. Stokes R. Letter: intestinal mycosis in a cat. Aust Vet J 1973;49(10):499-500.
33. Ascioglu S, Rex JH, de Pauw B, et al. Defining opportunistic invasive fungal infections in immunocompromised patients with cancer and hematopoietic stem cell transplants: an international consensus. Clin Infect Dis 2002;34(1): 7-14.
34. Segal BH. Medical progress aspergillosis. N Engl J Med 2009;360(18):1870-84.
35. Hope WW, Walsh TJ, Denning DW. The invasive and saprophytic syndromes due to Aspergillus spp. Med Mycol 2005;43:S207-38.
36. Chakrabarti A, Das A, Panda NK. Controversies surrounding the categorization of fungal sinusitis. Med Mycol 2009;47:S299-308.
37. Panda NK, Balaji P, Chakrabarti A, et al. Paranasal sinus aspergillosis: its categorization to develop a treatment protocol. Mycoses 2004;47(7):277-83.
38. Uri N, Cohen-Kerem R, Elmalah I, et al. Classification of fungal sinusitis in immunocompetent patients. Otolaryngol Head Neck Surg 2003;129(4):372-8.
39. Peeters D, Clercx C. Update on canine sinonasal aspergillosis. Vet Clin North Am Small Anim Pract 2007;37(5):901-16.
40. Malik R, Vogelnest L, O'Brien CR, et al. Infections and some other conditions affecting the skin and subcutis of the naso-ocular region of cats: clinical experience 1987-2003. J Feline Med Surg 2004;6(6):383-90.
41. Karnik K, Reichle JK, Fischetti AJ, et al. Computed tomographic findings of fungal rhinitis and sinusitis in cats. Vet Radiol Ultrasound 2009;50(1):65-8.
42. Furrow E, Groman RP. Intranasal infusion of clotrimazole for the treatment of nasal aspergillosis in two cats. J Am Vet Med Assoc 2009;235(10): 1188-93.
43. Barachetti L, Mortellaro CM, Di Giancamillo M, et al. Bilateral orbital and nasal aspergillosis in a cat. Vet Ophthalmol 2009;12(3):176-82.
44. Giordano C, Gianella P, Bo S, et al. Invasive mould infections of the naso-orbital region of cats: a case involving Aspergillus fumigatus and an aetiological review. J Feline Med Surg 2010;12(9):714-23.
45. Smith LN, Hoffman SB. A case series of unilateral orbital aspergillosis in three cats and treatment with voriconazole. Vet Ophthalmol 2010;13(3):190-203.
46. Schiefer B. Dtsch Tierarztl Wochenschr 1965;72:73.

47. Houbraken J, Samson RA. Phylogeny of penicillium and the segregation of Trichocomaceae into three families. Stud Mycol 2011;70:1–51.
48. Pomrantz JS, Johnson LR. Update on the efficacy of topical clotrimazole in the treatment of canine nasal aspergillosis. J Vet Intern Med 2007;21(3):608.
49. Pomrantz JS, Johnson LR. Repeated rhinoscopic and serologic assessment of the effectiveness of intranasally administered clotrimazole for the treatment of nasal aspergillosis in dogs. J Am Vet Med Assoc 2010;236(7):757–62.
50. Peeters D, Peters IR, Helps CR, et al. Whole blood and tissue fungal DNA quantification in the diagnosis of canine sinonasal aspergillosis. Vet Microbiol 2008; 128:194–203.
51. Balajee SA, Nickle D, Varga J, et al. Molecular studies reveal frequent misidentification of *Aspergillus fumigatus* by morphotyping. Eukaryot Cell 2006;5(10): 1705–12.
52. Balajee SA, Houbraken J, Verweij PE, et al. *Aspergillus* species identification in the clinical setting. Stud Mycol 2007;59:39–46.
53. Talbot J, Martin P, Johnson L, et al. What causes sino-nasal aspergillosis in dogs? A molecular approach to species identification. In: International Society of Infectious Diseases 2nd Symposium Proceedings, San Francisco, November 14–17, 2012. Abstract 018.
54. Varga J, Frisvad JC, Kocsube S, et al. New and revisited species in *Aspergillus* section Nigri. Stud Mycol 2011;69:1–17.
55. Samson RA, Hong S, Peterson SW, et al. Polyphasic taxonomy of *Aspergillus* section Fumigati and its teleomorph Neosartorya. Stud Mycol 2007;59:147–203.
56. Alcazar-Fuoli L, Mellado E, Aslastruey-Izquierdo A, et al. *Aspergillus* section fumigati: antifungal susceptibility patterns and sequence-based identification. Antimicrob Agents Chemother 2008;52(4):1244–51.
57. Pitt JI, Samson RA. Nomenclatural considerations in naming species of *Aspergillus* and its teleomorphs. Stud Mycol 2007;59:67–70.
58. O'Gorman CM, Fuller HT, Dyer PS. Discovery of a sexual cycle in the opportunistic fungal pathogen *Aspergillus fumigatus*. Nature 2009;457:471–4.
59. Miller JS, Funk VA, Wagner WL, et al. Outcomes of the 2011 botanical nomenclature section at the XVIII International Botanical Congress. PhytoKeys 2011; 5:1–3.
60. Hawksworth DL, Crous PW, Redhead SA, et al. The Amsterdam Declaration on fungal nomenclature. Mycotaxon 2011;116:491–500.
61. Sharp NJ, Harvey CE, Sullivan M. Canine nasal aspergillosis and penicilliosis. Compendium on Continuing Education for the Practicing Veterinarian 1991; 13(1):41–6.
62. Day MJ. Canine sino-nasal aspergillosis: parallels with human disease. Med Mycol 2009;47:S315–23.
63. Shoham S, Levitz SM. The immune response to fungal infections. Br J Haematol 2005;129(5):569–82.
64. Romani L. Immunity to fungal infections. Nat Rev Immunol 2011;11(4):275–88.
65. Gresnigt MS, Netea MG, van de Veerdonk FL. Pattern recognition receptors and their role in invasive aspergillosis. Ann N Y Acad Sci 2012;1273:60–7.
66. Peeters D, Peters IR, Clercx C, et al. Quantification of mRNA encoding cytokines and chemokines in nasal biopsies from dogs with sino-nasal aspergillosis. Vet Microbiol 2006;114(3–4):318–26.
67. Peeters D, Peters IR, Helps CR, et al. Distinct tissue cytokine and chemokine mRNA expression in canine sino-nasal aspergillosis and idiopathic lymphoplasmacytic rhinitis. Vet Immunol Immunopathol 2007;117(1–2):95–105.

68. Mercier E, Peters IR, Day MJ, et al. Toll- and NOD-like receptor mRNA expression in canine sino-nasal aspergillosis and idiopathic lymphoplasmacytic rhinitis. Vet Immunol Immunopathol 2012;145(3–4):618–24.
69. Vanherberghen M, Bureau F, Peters IR, et al. Analysis of gene expression in canine sino-nasal aspergillosis and idiopathic lymphoplasmacytic rhinitis: a transcriptomic analysis. Vet Microbiol 2012;157(1–2):143–51.
70. Romani L. Immunity to fungal infections. Nat Rev Immunol 2004;4(1):11–23.
71. Siddiqui AA, Shah AA, Bashir SH. Craniocerebral aspergillosis of sinonasal origin in immunocompetent patients: clinical spectrum and outcome in 25 cases. Neurosurgery 2004;55(3):602–11.
72. Latge JP. The pathobiology of *Aspergillus fumigatus*. Trends Microbiol 2001; 9(8):382–9.
73. Tomee JF, Kauffman HF. Putative virulence factors of *Aspergillus fumigatus*. Clin Exp Allergy 2000;30(4):476–84.
74. Sugui JA, Pardo J, Chang YC, et al. Gliotoxin is a virulence factor of *Aspergillus fumigatus*: gliP deletion attenuates virulence in mice immunosuppressed with hydrocortisone. Eukaryot Cell 2007;6(9):1562–9.
75. Hogan LH, Klein BS, Levitz SM. Virulence factors of medically important fungi. Clin Microbiol Rev 1996;9(4):469–87.
76. Barrs VR, Nicoll R, Beatty JA. Computed tomographic findings in 10 cases of feline upper respiratory aspergillosis. International Society for Companion Animal Infectious Diseases. 1st Symposium Proceedings, Toulouse, September 8–9, 2010.
77. Hope WW, Walsh TJ, Denning DW. Laboratory diagnosis of invasive aspergillosis. Lancet Infect Dis 2005;5:609–22.
78. Whitney J, Beatty JA, Dhand N, et al. Evaluation of serum galactomannan detection for the diagnosis of feline upper respiratory tract aspergillosis. Vet Microbiol 2013;162(1):5.
79. Hachem RY, Kontoyiannais DP, Chemaly RF, et al. Utility of galactomannan enzyme immunoassay and (1,3) B-D-glucan in diagnosis of invasive fungal infections: low sensitivity for *Aspergillus fumigatus* infection in hematologic malignancy patients. J Clin Microbiol 2009;47(1):129–33.
80. Pfeiffer CD, Fine JP, Safdar N. Diagnosis of invasive aspergillosis using a galactomannan assay: a meta-analysis. Clin Infect Dis 2006;42(10):1417–27.
81. Kitasato Y, Tao Y, Hoshino T, et al. Comparison of *Aspergillus* galactomannan antigen testing with a new cut-off index and *Aspergillus* precipitating antibody testing for the diagnosis of chronic pulmonary aspergillosis. Respirology 2009;14(5):701–8.
82. Mennink-Kersten M, Donnelly JP, Verweij PE. Detection of circulating galactomannan for the diagnosis and management of invasive aspergillosis. Lancet Infect Dis 2004;4(6):349–57.
83. Herbrecht R, Letscher-Bru V, Oprea C, et al. *Aspergillus* galactomannan detection in the diagnosis of invasive aspergillosis in cancer patients. J Clin Oncol 2002;20(7):1898–906.
84. Peeters D, Day MJ, Clercx C. An immunohistochemical study of canine nasal aspergillosis. J Comp Pathol 2005;132(4):283–8.
85. Siemann M, Koch-Dorfler M, Gaude M. False-positive results in premature infants with the Platelia (R) *Aspergillus* sandwich enzyme-linked immunosorbent assay. Mycoses 1998;41(9–10):373–7.
86. Zandijk E, Mewis A, Magerman K, et al. False-positive results by the platelia *Aspergillus* galactomannan antigen test for patients treated with amoxicillin-clavulanate. Clin Vaccine Immunol 2008;15(7):1132–3.

87. Lenglinger FX, Krennmair G, MullerSchelken H, et al. Radiodense concretions in maxillary sinus aspergillosis: pathogenesis and the role of CT densitometry. Eur Radiol 1996;6(3):375–9.
88. Tromblee TC, Jones JC, Etue AE, et al. Association between clinical characteristics, computed tomography characteristics, and histologic diagnosis for cats with sinonasal disease. Vet Radiol Ultrasound 2006;47(3):241–8.
89. Schoenborn WC, Wisner ER, Kass PP, et al. Retrospective assessment of computed tomographic imaging of feline sinonasal disease in 62 cats. Vet Radiol Ultrasound 2003;44(2):185–95.
90. Winstanley EW. Trephining frontal sinuses in the treatment of rhinitis and sinusitis in the cat. Vet Rec 1974;95:289–92.
91. Iwen PC, Hinrichs SH, Rupp ME. Utilization of the internal transcribed spacer regions as molecular targets to detect and identify human fungal pathogens. Med Mycol 2002;40(1):87–109.
92. Lau A, Chen S, Sorrell T, et al. Development and clinical application of a panfungal PCR assay to detect and identify fungal DNA in tissue specimens. J Clin Microbiol 2007;45(2):380–5.
93. Chen SC, Halliday CL, Meyer W. A review of nucleic acid-based diagnostic tests for systemic mycoses with an emphasis on polymerase chain reaction-based assays. Med Mycol 2002;40(4):333–57.
94. Samson RA, Varga J, Witiak SM, et al. The species concept in *Aspergillus*: recommendations of an international panel. Stud Mycol 2007;59:71–3.
95. Zonderland JL, Stork CK, Saunders JH, et al. Intranasal infusion of enilconazole for treatment of sinonasal aspergillosis in dogs. J Am Vet Med Assoc 2002; 221(10):1421–5.
96. Barr SC, Rishniw M, Lynch M. Questions contents of clotrimazole solution. J Am Vet Med Assoc 2010;236(2):163–4.
97. Quimby JM, Hoffman SB, Duke J, et al. Adverse neurologic events associated with voriconazole use in 3 cats. J Vet Intern Med 2010;24(3):647–9.
98. Walsh TJ, Anaissie EJ, Denning DW, et al. Treatment of aspergillosis: clinical practice guidelines of the Infectious Diseases Society of America. Clin Infect Dis 2008;46(3):327–60.

Canine Nasal Disease

Leah A. Cohn, DVM, PhD

KEYWORDS

- Rhinitis • Nasal discharge • Epistaxis • Sinonasal aspergillosis
- Nasal adenocarcinoma

KEY POINTS

- For dogs with epistaxis unaccompanied by mucoid or mucopurulent nasal discharge, assessment of coagulation status and blood pressure should precede diagnostic investigation aimed at identifying nasal disease.
- Investigation of oral health, including dental probing and dental radiographs as needed, is warranted before more expensive or invasive diagnostics are undertaken in dogs with nasal discharge.
- Primary bacterial rhinitis is uncommon as a cause of nasal disease signs, but antibiotics often result in temporary improvement in signs related to secondary bacterial infections.
- In retrospective studies, nasal neoplasia is often the most common cause of chronic nasal discharge or epistaxis in dogs.
- If the dog's owners are willing to undertake expensive therapies (eg, radiation therapy for nasal carcinoma), should they be indicated, computed tomography or magnetic resonance imaging is indicated early in the disease evaluation.

INTRODUCTION
Nature of the Problem

Canine nasal disease is commonly encountered in small animal practice. Clinical signs are similar regardless of the specific cause of nasal disease (**Box 1**), but some signs are more often associated with specific disease process (eg, facial deformity is more often identified in dogs with nasal neoplasia than other causes of nasal disease). In addition, nasal signs may be identified in dogs with systemic rather than nasal disease (**Box 2**).

A thorough history and physical examination, followed by a stepwise diagnostic evaluation, often identifies a specific diagnosis and thus facilitates an accurate prognosis and development of an optimum treatment plan. Several studies have described either a specific clinical disease that results in nasal signs,[1–7] or have described diagnostic modalities used in dogs with nasal signs.[8–14] Only a few

Department of Veterinary Medicine and Surgery, University of Missouri, 900 East Campus Drive, Columbia, MO 65211, USA
E-mail address: cohnl@missouri.edu

Vet Clin Small Anim 44 (2014) 75–89
http://dx.doi.org/10.1016/j.cvsm.2013.08.002   vetsmall.theclinics.com
0195-5616/14/$ – see front matter © 2014 Elsevier Inc. All rights reserved.

Box 1
Clinical signs associated with canine nasal disease

Nasal discharge

  Serous

  Mucoid

  Mucopurulent

  Purulent

  Sanguineus/epistaxis

  Mixed

Sneezing

Pawing or rubbing at muzzle

Facial deformity, asymmetry, or ulceration

Epiphora

Loss of pigmentation of the nasal planum

Open mouth breathing

Halitosis

Stertor

Coughing

Seizure (rare)

---

retrospective studies have investigated the frequency with which specific diagnosis is determined to cause nasal signs in dogs.[15–18] Understanding which diagnoses are most likely is helpful not only in prioritizing diagnostic testing but also in informing pet owners as they consider which of many diagnostic options to authorize. Retrospective studies undertaken at referral institutions might provide a biased representation of the relative importance of some conditions because many common disorders could be treated by local veterinarians without need for referral. Nonetheless, retrospective studies provide useful information regarding the most common causes of nasal disease (**Fig. 1**).

Box 2
Systemic diseases processes with nasal manifestations

Coagulopathy

  Primary hemostatic defects (ie, thrombocytopenia/thrombocytopathia)

  Secondary hemostatic defects (eg, vitamin K rodenticide antagonists)

Severe hypertension

Hyperviscosity syndromes (eg, multiple myeloma, ehrlichiosis)

Systemic infection (eg, distemper virus)

Dysautonomia

Vomiting/regurgitation

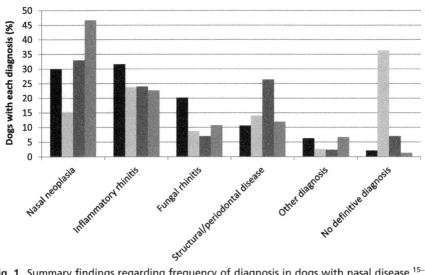

Fig. 1. Summary findings regarding frequency of diagnosis in dogs with nasal disease.[15–18] Although each study classified disease diagnosis differently, diagnoses have been grouped similarly for summary presentation. (*Data from* Refs.[15–18])

CLINICAL FINDINGS
History and Signalment

Nasal disease occurs most often in doliocephalic and mesocephalic dogs.[13,15–17] In particular, doliocephalic breeds are 2.5 times more likely to develop nasal neoplasia than are mixed breed dogs, and large dogs are more likely to have nasal neoplasia than small breeds.[19–21] Although some studies suggest a slight overrepresentation of male dogs for nasal neoplasia, other studies find no relationship between sex and various causes of nasal disease.[13,15–18,21] There are relationships between the age of the dog and disease. Nasal neoplasia, one of the most common causes of nasal discharge and epistaxis, is more likely in older dogs.[13,16,17,22] Similarly, periodontal disease is more likely in older dogs. Inflammatory rhinitis occurs in dogs of all ages.[4,13,18] Although it can also occur in dogs of any age, fungal rhinitis is most often recognized in young to middle-aged adults.[23]

History provided by the dog's owners can be useful. Key questions include:

- Are there signs of illness that are not directly related to the nose, such as anorexia, weight loss, lethargy, bleeding, or bruising?
- What is the duration of nasal signs, and have any therapies been attempted? If so, what was the response?
- Did the dog's environment change before the clinical signs began (including trips to a boarding facility or a move to a new location)?
- If nasal discharge is present, does it come from 1 nostril (and if so, which one) or both? Has discharge changed from unilateral to bilateral?
- What is the predominant character of nasal discharge, and has it changed over time?
- If nasal signs are long-standing, is there a seasonal change?

Acute nasal signs, nasal signs associated with systemic illness, and epistaxis in the absence of other nasal signs should prompt a thorough consideration of nonnasal disease. For dogs with an acute onset of mucopurulent or purulent discharge, serious consideration should be given to systemic infection (eg distemper, influenza virus) rather than local nasal disease. Although causes of epistaxis directly related to disease of the nose are identified at least 3 times more frequently than are systemic causes of epistaxis, it is still crucial that systemic disorders be ruled out before beginning a search for nasal disease.[24] For dogs presenting with epistaxis in the absence of mucoid/purulent/mucopurulent nasal discharge, coagulation disorders, hypertension, or hyperviscosity syndromes must be ruled out before undertaking nasal imaging or biopsy.

Duration of signs influences the likelihood of various diagnoses. Nasal foreign bodies often result in an acute onset of sneezing and facial pawing, but can remain in place for a long period, resulting in chronic nasal discharge. Signs related to nasal neoplasia or fungal rhinitis can be present for days, weeks, or even months before presentation.[20] However, if signs are present for many months without disease progression, cancer and fungal rhinitis become less likely, whereas structural (eg, nasal stenosis, oronasal fistulae) or inflammatory disease becomes more likely. Seasonal variation in severity of signs is suggestive of inflammatory rather than structural disease.

Laterality of nasal discharge can provide clues to the cause of nasal signs.[15,18] Nasal discharge associated with nasal foreign bodies or structural defects is generally unilateral. Discharge associated with either nasal neoplasia or fungal rhinitis often begins as a unilateral problem but progresses to bilateral involvement. Although nasal discharge associated with periodontal disease is often unilateral, dogs with poor oral health can have problems on both sides of the mouth and therefore could show bilateral nasal discharge. Inflammatory rhinitis can present with either unilateral or bilateral nasal discharge.[4]

Response to previous therapy with either antihistamines or antibiotics does not necessarily incriminate primary allergic or infectious disease, respectively. Antihistamines can result in minor improvement, regardless of disease causation. Similarly, antibiotic therapy can change the quality or quantity of nasal discharge either through elimination of secondary, opportunistic bacterial pathogens or via an antiinflammatory effect (as seen with doxycycline[25]), regardless of the underlying disease process.

Physical Examination

Physical examination can be useful in establishing and prioritizing differential diagnosis. In addition to an examination of the head, examination of the entire dog is warranted. For animals with epistaxis, look carefully for petechia or ecchymosis, which suggest coagulopathy. Retinal examination might reveal evidence of either coagulopathy or hypertension. Specific examination should include each of the following:

- Symmetry of the face and muzzle
- Character of nasal discharge, with notation of side(s)
- Facial deformity or ulceration
- Patency of airflow through each nostril
- Condition of the teeth and gums
- Examination of the roof of the mouth to the pharynx (to degree possible)
- Ability to retropulse the eyes
- Pain on opening the mouth or manipulating the muzzle
- Epiphora
- Percussion of the frontal sinuses and muzzle
- Pigmentation of the nasal planum
- Size and texture of submandibular lymph nodes

A thorough evaluation of the oral cavity includes probing the sulci around the teeth because disease can be present beneath the gum line. Because this examination requires heavy sedation or anesthesia, it is often completed just before, or immediately after, imaging studies or other diagnostic examinations. If probing reveals periodontal disease before advanced imaging is performed, it might obviate that expensive testing. On the other hand, bleeding that can occur as a result of periodontal probing can negatively affect subsequent imaging studies. Therefore, the clinician must use their best judgment in deciding if periodontal probing should precede or follow imaging studies. Tooth root abscess, oronasal fistulae, fractured teeth, osteomyelitis, and intranasal migration of displaced teeth are all potential causes of nasal discharge. Often, dental radiographs are beneficial, especially when disease of a specific tooth is suspected.

Although physical examination rarely provides a definitive diagnosis unless periodontal disease is identified, it often allows for a logical rank order for differential diagnosis. Deformity of the face, epiphora, inability to retropulse the eyes, or ulceration on the muzzle itself often suggest space-occupying neoplastic disease.[15] Loss of pigment on the nasal planum suggests sinonasal aspergillosis,[23] whereas ulcers of the nasal planum can be either fungal or neoplastic in origin. Absence of airflow suggests a space-occupying lesion, although severe mucus accumulation or a foreign body can produce the same effect.[17]

Nasal discharge can be characterized as either serous, mucoid, purulent, hemorrhagic, or some combination of those types. Although character of the discharge cannot be used to make a diagnosis, certain differential diagnoses are more or less likely to be associated with certain types of discharge (**Box 3**).[13,18] Any nasal disease that disrupts the normal protective mechanisms can result in secondary bacterial infection and associated purulent discharge, making this (the most common type of discharge) perhaps the least useful in ranking differential diagnosis lists.

DIAGNOSTIC MODALITIES

Choice of diagnostic modalities depends on a logically ordered list of differential diagnoses, availability of equipment, and the wishes of the animal's owner (a factor often related to cost). Certain diagnostic techniques can be low yield, but because of simplicity and low cost are still worthwhile. As an example, metastasis of nasal neoplasia to the submandibular lymph nodes at disease diagnosis is uncommon ($\sim 8\%$), but fine-needle aspirate of those nodes is simple, inexpensive, minimally invasive, and can occasionally provide a definitive disease diagnosis.[22]

Box 3
Characteristics of nasal discharge associated with disease causation

• Serous discharge

Consider: nasal mites, allergy, early viral infection, stress.

• Mucoid or mucopurulent discharge

Consider: systemic disease, oronasal/periodontal disease, nasal neoplasia, inflammatory nasal disease (reactive or primary), fungal rhinitis, foreign body, secondary bacterial infection.

• Epistaxis

Consider: systemic disease, trauma, nasal neoplasia, fungal rhinitis, inflammatory nasal disease.

Imaging Studies

Imaging studies are useful for the diagnosis of nasal disease in dogs. These studies include:

- Dental radiographs (as indicated based on oral examination)
- Skull radiographs
- Thoracic radiographs
- Computed tomography (CT) of the skull with or without contrast enhancement
- Magnetic resonance imaging (MRI) of the skull
- Rhinoscopy, including choanal examination

The usefulness of thoracic radiographs is debatable, because most nasal tumors are locally invasive and unlikely to metastasize to the lungs. However, thoracic imaging is a reasonable diagnostic technique for dogs with suspected nasal neoplasia, because recognition of metastasis likely alters diagnostic and therapeutic plans. When both radiographic/CT/MRI imaging of the nose and rhinoscopy are planned, radiographic studies should always precede rhinoscopy, because rhinoscopy results in hemorrhage, which can alter results of radiographic studies.

Numerous studies have described the usefulness of plain film nasal radiographs, CT, and MRI in the diagnosis of nasal disease.[10,12–14,22,26,27] Advantages and disadvantages exist with each modality (**Table 1**). Appropriate plain film nasal radiographs require multiple views, including open mouth views, and thus require general anesthesia. Although either CT or MRI provides significant additional information and increases diagnostic sensitivity in dogs with nasal disease compared with plain radiographs, cost and availability are limitations for some pet owners. However, for pet owners who are likely to consider definitive forms of therapy (eg, radiation for nasal neoplasia or intranasal instillation of antifungal drugs for the treatment of sinonasal aspergillosis), the advantages of advanced imaging are great enough that early referral to an institution with these capabilities is warranted. Although imaging cannot provide a histopathologic diagnosis, advanced imaging can often provide a good degree of confidence in a probable diagnosis.

Rhinoscopy allows direct visualization of the nasal passages and, via a retroflexed view using a flexible scope, the choanae.[28–30] Rhinoscopy is most useful in

		Skull Radiographs	CT	MRI
Table 1				
Comparison of imaging techniques for dogs with nasal disease				
Availability		Readily available	Moderate availability	Least available
General anesthesia		Required	Anesthesia or sedation	Required
Cost		Least expensive	Moderately expensive	Most expensive
Show cribriform plate integrity		Poor	Excellent	Excellent
Ability to discriminate between tissue and mucus		Poor	Excellent (with contrast)	Excellent
Sensitivity to detect soft tissue changes		Poor to moderate	Good	Excellent
Sensitivity to detect bony changes (lysis or hyperostosis)		Moderate	Excellent	Good
Ability to evaluate sinuses		Moderate	Excellent	Good to excellent

combination with, and immediately after, radiographic imaging. Visualization of nasal mites, foreign materials, fungal plaques, or stenosis/atresia can provide a specific diagnosis (**Fig. 2**). Destruction of nasal turbinates in dogs with sinonasal aspergillosis can create a characteristic cavernous appearance with or without visible fungal plaques. Tumors often block passage of the scope, but malignancy cannot be confirmed by rhinoscopic appearance alone. Hyperemia, mucus, and blood are frequently identified but nonspecific abnormalities. In addition to viewing lesions, rhinoscopy can be used to guide tissue biopsy.[28]

Nonimaging Diagnostic Modalities

Besides diagnostic modalities used to rule out systemic causes of nasal signs (eg, blood pressure measurement, coagulation assays), there are a variety of non–imaging-related diagnostic modalities that are useful for animals with nasal disease. Some are applied in nearly all animals with nasal disease (eg, probing of the dental sulci), whereas others are reserved for use in only select cases (eg, fungal serology or culture). Nonimaging diagnostic modalities include:

- Dental probing under sedation/anesthesia
    A simple, noninvasive technique applied to essentially all dogs with chronic nasal signs. Dental probe examination has a high diagnostic yield when signs are related to oral/periodontal disease.

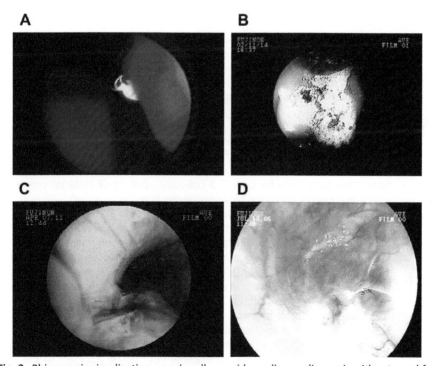

Fig. 2. Rhinoscopic visualization occasionally provides a disease diagnosis without need for additional testing. (*A*) A nasal mite seen in a dog presented for sneezing and pawing at the nose. (*B*) A fungal plaque in a dog with nasal aspergillosis. (*C*) A grass foreign body associated with an acute onset of sneezing. (*D*) Nasopharyngeal stenosis observed on a retroflexed view to the choane. (*Courtesy of* [*A*] Dr Carol Reinero, DVM, PhD, DACVIM (SAIM), Columbia, MO; and [*C*] Dr Laura Nafe, DVM, MS, DACVIM (SAIM), Columbia, MO.)

- Serology

  Noninvasive blood tests (agar-gel immunodiffusion or IgG enzyme-linked immunosorbent assay) provide good sensitivity and excellent specificity for sinonasal aspergillosis, but serum/urine galactomannan assays are of no value.[31,32] Serologic tests are best used when aspergillosis is suspected based on clinical findings but either pet owners have declined more expensive diagnostic techniques (ie, advanced imaging studies), or when infection could not be confirmed by other methods. Latex agglutination titers for nasal cryptococcosis provide good sensitivity and specificity, but nasal cryptococcosis is less common in dogs than in cats.

- Fine-needle aspirate of submandibular lymph nodes

  The diagnostic yield of this simple, noninvasive technique is low, because metastasis at time of disease diagnosis is uncommon. Submandibular lymph nodes that are enlarged, firm, or ipsilateral to suspected nasal neoplasia warrant aspirate with cytology despite low sensitivity.[20–22]

- Nasal cytology

  Cytologic assessment of impressions from biopsy specimens, nasal swabs or brush samples (collected with or without visual guidance), or nasal discharge are, respectively, more or less useful for disease diagnosis. Disease diagnosis based on cytologic assessment of nasal discharge is unlikely, but guided sampling can provide higher diagnostic yield if disease is caused by neoplasia or fungal infection.[16,33]

- Nasal fungal culture

  Fungal cultures require substantial time for pathogen growth and are not inexpensive. The sensitivity of culture for dogs with sinonasal aspergillosis can be as high as 80% if samples are collected from areas containing rhinoscopically visible plaques, but are likely lower from randomly obtained samples.[31] It can be argued that fungal culture is not necessary if fungal plaques are visualized.

- Nasal bacterial culture

  Because the nasal passages of healthy dogs are not sterile, and because primary bacterial rhinitis is rare, I find little use for bacterial culture from dogs with nasal disease. Culture collection method likely influences culture results from dogs as it does for cats.[34] If collected, culture of material (tissue or swab) from deep within the nasal passages is recommended.

- Nasal biopsy with histopathologic evaluation

  Although an invasive technique that requires general anesthesia, biopsy is typically required for a definitive diagnosis. It is the only means to confirm a diagnosis of inflammatory rhinitis, including lymphoplasmacytic rhinitis.[4] Histopathologic examination of biopsy tissue can identify fungal pathogens or confirm a specific type of nasal neoplasia.[21] Biopsy techniques include rhinoscopically guided biopsy, biopsy guided by radiographic imaging, blind biopsy, or nasal hydropulsion.[30,35,36] Care must be used in obtaining biopsy without visual guidance (**Fig. 3**). Especially when conducted in a blinded fashion, sampling can miss the lesion and provide misleading information, because of collection of material from tissue adjacent to the primary lesion.

- Nasal lavage

  Nasal lavage/hydropulsion can be used as a diagnostic tool in anesthetized dogs. It is most useful either when used to dislodge tumor tissue for histopathologic examination, or when used to dislodge foreign material (eg, plant

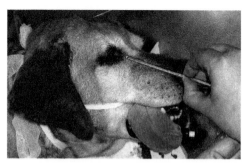

Fig. 3. Preparation for blinded nasal biopsy. The biopsy instrument should be measured against the distance from the nares to the medial canthus of the eye before biopsy in order to avoid penetration of the central nervous system.

material).[35] Cytologic evaluation or culture of the lavage solution can occasionally allow identification of fungal hyphae or neoplastic cells.

- Rhinotomy/sinusotomy/frontal sinus trephination

    This most invasive option for diagnosis of nasal disease is usually reserved for those cases that elude diagnosis using other techniques. Although CT or MRI might strongly suggest a diagnosis of sinonasal aspergillosis, confirmation by rhinoscopic visualization of fungal plaques in the nasal cavity or fungal culture is not always possible.[7] In these cases, surgical access to the sinuses can both confirm a diagnosis and facilitate treatment. Similarly, neoplastic disease is sometimes best accessed through a surgical approach when other methods have failed to yield a diagnosis. However, surgical debulking of nasal neoplasia is not curative, with radiation therapy generally the preferred option for treatment with or without surgical exoneration.[37,38]

PATHOLOGY

Confirmation of tumor type depends on histopathologic evaluation of nasal tissue. In dogs, carcinoma accounts for as much as two-thirds of nasal neoplasia, with adenocarcinoma the most common tumor type (**Box 4**).

Pathologic assessment of tissue biopsy is also necessary for diagnosis of inflammatory nasal disease. Diagnosis of inflammatory nasal disease is often frustrating both because of the lack of any specific findings other than histopathologic changes and because these same histopathologic changes can be identified in dogs with other types of nasal disease. Idiopathic lymphoplasmacytic inflammation is the most commonly identified inflammatory rhinitis, but suppurative rhinitis, eosinophilic rhinitis, and granulomatous rhinitis occur as well.[13] Clinicians must keep in mind that inflammation can reflect a response to disease rather than the disease itself. For example, nasal discharge can occur in animals with vomiting or regurgitation as a result of aspiration of materials into the choanae or caudal nasal passage (**Fig. 4**); tissue biopsy from these dogs shows inflammation on microscopic examination, but not disease causation. In addition, biopsy samples can miss the underlying disease and show only surrounding inflammation. When biopsy identifies only inflammation, but neoplastic or fungal rhinitis are suspected based on clinical signs or imaging results, either alternative diagnostic testing (eg, fungal serology) or more aggressive repeat biopsy (eg, rhinotomy) may be warranted.

Box 4
Canine nasal neoplasia

Most commonly identified nasal tumor types

- Adenocarcinoma
- Undifferentiated carcinoma
- Chondrosarcoma
- Squamous cell carcinoma

Occasionally identified nasal tumor types

- Fibrosarcoma
- Osteosarcoma
- Undifferentiated sarcoma
- Lymphoma

Rarely identified nasal tumor types (other types are possible)

- Melanoma
- Hemangiosarcoma
- Transmissible venereal tumor
- Neuroendocrine carcinoma
- Mast cell tumors

Data from Refs.[13,20,39,40]

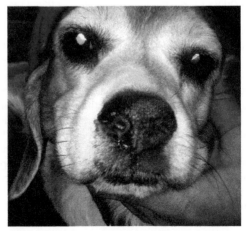

Fig. 4. Severe mucopurulent nasal discharge caused by inflammation of the nasal cavity induced by severe persistent vomiting in a dog with pancreatitis.

CASE STUDIES
Case Study 1

A five-year-old female spayed (FS) Siberian husky presented for an episode of severe epistaxis.

History
Although the dog presented for acute epistaxis, its owners acknowledged that mucopurulent nasal discharge had been present for 2 to 3 weeks; they were unsure as to which side(s) had been affected.

Physical examination
Temperature, pulse, and respiration were normal. Examination (including ocular and conscious oral examination) was unremarkable save for bilateral mucopurulent discharge, with some blood from the right nostril and loss of pigmentation on the nasal planum (**Fig. 5**). The dog resented manipulation of the muzzle. Patent airflow was present from both nares.

Diagnostic evaluation
The combination of epistaxis with mucopurulent discharge, and the absence of petechia or ecchymosis, made systemic disease (eg, coagulopathy, hypertension) less likely than nasal disease. Patent airflow, pain on manipulation of the muzzle, and loss of pigmentation brought nasal aspergillosis to the top of the differential list, which still included periodontal disease, nasal neoplasia, inflammatory nasal disease, or foreign body.

Under general anesthesia, a thorough oral examination with dental probing did not identify important periodontal disease. CT showed cavitary destruction of the turbinates as well as loss of nasal septal bone and mucosal thickening; the cribriform plate was intact. Rhinoscopy, completed after CT examination, showed loss of nasal turbinates, mucoid/sanguinous nasal discharge, and multiple white plaques typical of sinonasal aspergillosis. Fungal culture was not obtained, but samples were submitted for histopathologic examination and later confirmed the presence of fungal elements. The combination of clinical and diagnostic findings provided enough confidence in the diagnosis of fungal rhinitis to warrant treatment during the same anesthetic episode as the diagnostic testing. The nasal cavity was debrided and treated with installation of enilconazole.[23] The dog made a complete recovery and did not require subsequent repeated therapy.

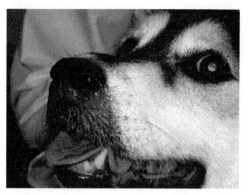

Fig. 5. Five-year-old FS Siberian husky presented for epistaxis. Notice mucopurulent nasal discharge and loss of pigmentation on nasal planum. The diagnosis was nasal aspergillosis.

Case Study 2

An 11-year-old male catrated (MC) Labrador retriever presented for epistaxis.

History

The dog had a month-long history of sneezing unresponsive to antihistamines, glucocorticoids, or antibiotics, and was referred for diagnostic testing after an acute episode of epistaxis from the left nostril. Other than the recent nose bleed, no other discharge had been noticed.

Physical examination

Temperature was 41.1°C (103°F) and the dog was panting on initial examination. Facial asymmetry was present, with swelling under the left eye, elevation of the nictitans on the left, and inability to retropulse the left eye; the dog acted as if in pain when retropulsion was attempted. Airflow was absent through the left nasal passages. The left submandibular lymph node was slightly firm and enlarged. The remainder of the examination was unremarkable except for 2 movable subcutaneous masses on the flank.

Diagnostic evaluation

The combination of epistaxis with sneezing, facial asymmetry, and obstructed airflow pointed toward nasal rather than systemic disease. Facial asymmetry and absence of airflow on the left side of the face suggested a space-occupying lesion, and nasal neoplasia rose to the top of the differential diagnosis list.

The dog's owner was unsure if he would be willing to treat neoplastic disease should that be the final diagnosis. With this in mind, evaluation began with fine-needle aspirate of the left submandibular node; aspirate was nondiagnostic. Thoracic radiographs were offered to check for metastasis, but were declined because of the low likelihood of identifying metastatic nasal disease. The owner did agree to allow blind nasal biopsy. Biopsy revealed only lymphoplasmacytic rhinitis.

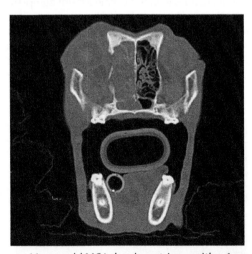

Fig. 6. CT image from an 11-year-old MC Labrador retriever with a 1-month history of sneezing and acute-onset epistaxis. The entire left nasal cavity was filled with contrast-enhancing soft tissue, with widespread destruction of the nasal turbinates. Multifocal lysis of the medial aspect of the left orbit with extension of the nasal mass into the medial aspect of the orbit was identified, with mild exophthalmos on the left. Findings were strongly suggestive of nasal neoplasia, which was confirmed on histopathology.

One week later, the dog's owner decided to pursue CT imaging (**Fig. 6**). Images were strongly suggestive of nasal neoplasia, with a contrast-enhancing space-occupying mass, substantial bony destruction, and enlargement of the regional lymph node. Repeat biopsies were obtained with guidance provided by the CT images, and the histopathologic diagnosis was nasal adenocarcinoma. The owner opted against radiation therapy.

SUMMARY

Nasal disease is a common problem in dogs, most often manifest as nasal discharge with or without other nasal signs. Attention to signalment, history, and physical examination findings often allows development of a logically ordered list of differential diagnosis. Once systemic and oral/periodontal disease have been ruled out, a combination of imaging techniques and tissue sampling for microscopic examination is usually necessary to achieve a diagnosis. Advanced imaging such as CT or MRI offers important advantages over traditional skull radiographs but are less widely available and more costly. Bacterial culture is seldom beneficial, and fungal culture is reserved for cases likely to have fungal rhinitis. Nasal biopsy is required to confirm a specific diagnosis and is always required for diagnosis of specific tumor type or for inflammatory rhinitis.

REFERENCES

1. Madewell BR, Priester WA, Gillette EL, et al. Neoplasms of the nasal passages and paranasal sinuses in domesticated animals as reported by 13 veterinary colleges. Am J Vet Res 1976;37(7):851–6.
2. MacEwen EG, Withrow SJ, Patnaik AK. Nasal tumors in the dog: retrospective evaluation of diagnosis, prognosis, and treatment. J Am Vet Med Assoc 1977; 170(1):45–8.
3. Van Pelt DR, McKiernan BC. Pathogenesis and treatment of canine rhinitis. Vet Clin North Am Small Anim Pract 1994;24(5):789–806.
4. Windsor RC, Johnson LR, Herrgesell EJ, et al. Idiopathic lymphoplasmacytic rhinitis in dogs: 37 cases (1997-2002). J Am Vet Med Assoc 2004;224(12):1952–7.
5. Windsor RC, Johnson LR, Sykes JE, et al. Molecular detection of microbes in nasal tissue of dogs with idiopathic lymphoplasmacytic rhinitis. J Vet Intern Med 2006;20(2):250–6.
6. Windsor RC, Johnson LR. Canine chronic inflammatory rhinitis. Clin Tech Small Anim Pract 2006;21(2):76–81.
7. Johnson LR, Drazenovich TL, Herrera MA, et al. Results of rhinoscopy alone or in conjunction with sinuscopy in dogs with aspergillosis: 46 cases (2001-2004). J Am Vet Med Assoc 2006;228(5):738–42.
8. Park RD, Beck ER, LeCouteur RA. Comparison of computed tomography and radiography for detecting changes induced by malignant nasal neoplasia in dogs. J Am Vet Med Assoc 1992;201:1720–4.
9. Burk RL. Computed tomographic imaging of nasal disease in 100 dogs. Vet Radiol Ultrasound 1992;33:177–80.
10. Codner EC, Lurus AG, Miller JB, et al. Comparison of computed tomography with radiography as a noninvasive diagnostic technique for chronic nasal disease in dogs. J Am Vet Med Assoc 1993;202(7):1106–10.
11. Saunders JH, van Bree H, Gielen I, et al. Diagnostic value of computed tomography in dogs with chronic nasal disease. Vet Radiol Ultrasound 2003;44(4):409–13.

12. Saunders JH, van Bree H. Comparison of radiography and computed tomography for the diagnosis of canine nasal aspergillosis. Vet Radiol Ultrasound 2003; 44(4):414–9.

13. Lefebvre J, Kuehn NF, Wortinger A. Computed tomography as an aid in the diagnosis of chronic nasal disease in dogs. J Small Anim Pract 2005;46(6): 280–5.

14. Miles MS, Dhaliwal RS, Moore MP, et al. Association of magnetic resonance imaging findings and histologic diagnosis in dogs with nasal disease: 78 cases (2001-2004). J Am Vet Med Assoc 2008;232(12):1844–9.

15. Lobetti RG. A retrospective study of chronic nasal disease in 75 dogs. J S Afr Vet Assoc 2009;80(4):224–8.

16. Meler E, Dunn M, Lecuyer M. A retrospective study of canine persistent nasal disease: 80 cases (1998-2003). Can Vet J 2008;49(1):71–6.

17. Tasker S, Knottenbelt CM, Munro EA, et al. Aetiology and diagnosis of persistent nasal disease in the dog: a retrospective study of 42 cases. J Small Anim Pract 1999;40(10):473–8.

18. Bondy PJ Jr, Cohn LA. Retrospective review of chronic nasal discharge in the dog [abstract]. J Vet Intern Med 2003;17:386.

19. Reif JS, Bruns C, Lower KS. Cancer of the nasal cavity and paranasal sinuses and exposure to environmental tobacco smoke in pet dogs. Am J Epidemiol 1998;147(5):488–92.

20. LaDue TA, Dodge R, Page RL, et al. Factors influencing survival after radiotherapy of nasal tumors in 130 dogs. Vet Radiol Ultrasound 1999;40(3):312–7.

21. Malinowski C. Canine and feline nasal neoplasia. Clin Tech Small Anim Pract 2006;21(2):89–94.

22. Avner A, Dobson JM, Sales JI, et al. Retrospective review of 50 canine nasal tumours evaluated by low-field magnetic resonance imaging. J Small Anim Pract 2008;49:233–9.

23. Sharman MJ, Mansfield CS. Sinonasal aspergillosis in dogs: a review. J Small Anim Pract 2012;53(8):434–44.

24. Bissett SA, Drobatz KJ, McKnight A, et al. Prevalence, clinical features, and causes of epistaxis in dogs: 176 cases (1996-2001). J Am Vet Med Assoc 2007;231(12):1843–50.

25. Leite LM, Carvalho AG, Ferreira PL, et al. Anti-inflammatory properties of doxycycline and minocycline in experimental models: an in vivo and in vitro comparative study. Inflammopharmacology 2011;19(2):99–110.

26. Saunders JH, Clercx C, Snaps FR, et al. Radiographic, magnetic resonance imaging, computed tomographic, and rhinoscopic features of nasal aspergillosis in dogs. J Am Vet Med Assoc 2004;225(11):1703–12.

27. Johnson EG, Wisner ER. Advances in respiratory imaging. Vet Clin North Am Small Anim Pract 2007;37(5):879–900, vi.

28. Lent SE, Hawkins EC. Evaluation of rhinoscopy and rhinoscopy-assisted mucosal biopsy in diagnosis of nasal disease in dogs: 119 cases (1985-1989). J Am Vet Med Assoc 1992;201(9):1425–9.

29. Willard MD, Radlinsky MA. Endoscopic examination of the choanae in dogs and cats: 118 cases (1988-1998). J Am Vet Med Assoc 1999;215(9):1301–5.

30. Elie M, Sabo M. Basics in canine and feline rhinoscopy. Clin Tech Small Anim Pract 2006;21(2):60–3.

31. Pomrantz JS, Johnson LR, Nelson RW, et al. Comparison of serologic evaluation via agar gel immunodiffusion and fungal culture of tissue for diagnosis of nasal aspergillosis in dogs. J Am Vet Med Assoc 2007;230(9):1319–23.

32. Billen F, Peeters D, Peters IR, et al. Comparison of the value of measurement of serum galactomannan and *Aspergillus*-specific antibodies in the diagnosis of canine sino-nasal aspergillosis. Vet Microbiol 2009;133(4):358–65.
33. De Lorenzi D, Bonfanti U, Masserdotti C, et al. Diagnosis of canine nasal aspergillosis by cytological examination: a comparison of four different collection techniques. J Small Anim Pract 2006;47(6):316–9.
34. Johnson LR, Kass PH. Effect of sample collection methodology on nasal culture results in cats. J Feline Med Surg 2009;11(8):645–9.
35. Ashbaugh EA, McKiernan BC, Miller CJ, et al. Nasal hydropulsion: a novel tumor biopsy technique. J Am Anim Hosp Assoc 2011;47(5):312–6.
36. Sapierzynski R, Zmudzka M. Endoscopy and histopathology in the examination of the nasal cavity in dogs. Pol J Vet Sci 2009;12(2):195–201.
37. Adams WM, Bjorling DE, McAnulty JE, et al. Outcome of accelerated radiotherapy alone or accelerated radiotherapy followed by exenteration of the nasal cavity in dogs with intranasal neoplasia: 53 cases (1990-2002). J Am Vet Med Assoc 2005;227(6):936–41.
38. Tan-Coleman B, Lyons J, Lewis C, et al. Prospective evaluation of a 5 × 4 Gy prescription for palliation of canine nasal tumors. Vet Radiol Ultrasound 2013;54(1): 89–92.
39. Rogers KS, Walker MA, Dillon HB. Transmissible venereal tumor: a retrospective study of 29 cases. J Am Anim Hosp Assoc 1998;34:463–70.
40. Adams WM, Kleiter MM, Thrall DE, et al. Prognostic significance of tumor histology and computed tomographic staging for radiation treatment response of canine nasal tumors. Vet Radiol Ultrasound 2009;50(3):330–5.

Update on Feline Asthma

Julie E. Trzil, DVM, Carol R. Reinero, DVM, PhD*

KEYWORDS

- Feline asthma • Feline lower airway disease • Airway eosinophilia
- Airway hyperresponsiveness

KEY POINTS

- Feline asthma is an important chronic lower airway disease of cats; however, definitive diagnosis is challenging because of overlapping clinicopathologic features with other lower airway disorders.
- Discriminating asthma from other chronic lower airway diseases (eg, infectious or chronic bronchitis or a variety of parasitic infections) is necessary because of differences in pathogenesis, novel treatments, and prognosis.
- Emerging diagnostics including thoracic CT scans and pulmonary function testing may help differentiate feline asthma from other chronic lower airway diseases.
- Therapy for feline asthma using glucocorticoids and bronchodilators might be inadequate or contraindicated in some cats; novel treatments investigated in experimental models of feline asthma could be beneficial in refractory cases or as adjuncts for glucocorticoid-sparing effects.

INTRODUCTION

Asthma is a common lower airway inflammatory disease in cats thought to be allergic in cause.[1] It is most commonly treated with glucocorticoids and bronchodilators. Although these are effective treatments in many cats, some cats are unresponsive or minimally responsive. In addition, chronic glucocorticoid therapy might not be well tolerated or could be contraindicated with certain diseases, such as diabetes mellitus or congestive heart failure. Finally, these therapies fail to reverse the abnormal immune response and ultimately do not ameliorate chronic airway remodeling that results in declining lung function. New therapies capable of restoring immune tolerance, acting more selectively to diminish allergic immune dysfunction with minimal systemic effects, or blunting airway remodeling would be desirable. Evaluation of novel

Funding Sources: None.
Conflict of Interest: None.
Comparative Internal Medicine Laboratory, Department of Veterinary Medicine and Surgery, College of Veterinary Medicine, University of Missouri, 900 East Campus Drive, Columbia, MO 65211, USA
* Corresponding author.
E-mail address: reineroc@missouri.edu

therapeutics in clinical trials of pet cats with asthma is hindered by a lack of consensus on what defines asthma and how it can be discriminated from other lower airway disorders. Thus, development of additional diagnostic tests in this arena is sorely needed. This article reviews what is currently known regarding the diagnosis and treatment of feline asthma as well as several new diagnostics and treatments that are on the horizon.

EPIDEMIOLOGY

Defining epidemiologic factors in feline asthma is complicated by a lack of consensus regarding what defines asthma in cats and how in practice it is best discriminated from other disorders. Most published studies fail to discriminate spontaneous feline asthma from chronic bronchitis, combining information from both disorders. Feline asthma is estimated to affect approximately 1% to 5% of the feline population.[2] Although the median age at presentation is 4 to 5 years, many cats have a history of chronic signs, suggesting that disease onset occurs much earlier in life.[3–5] There is no clear gender predilection.[3–7] The Siamese breed is overrepresented in some studies,[3,7] but not others.[4,6]

PATHOGENESIS

Evidence that asthma is mediated by an allergic response after exposure to inhaled aeroallergens is reviewed in detail elsewhere.[1] Aeroallergen-induced stimulation of a T helper 2 response leads to elaboration of a variety of cytokines. These cytokines drive the molecular switches that lead to pathologic changes in the airways. The 3 major hallmark features of asthma extrapolated from the disease in humans include airway inflammation, airway hyperresponsiveness and airflow limitation (the latter being at least in part reversible), and airway remodeling.[8]

PATIENT HISTORY AND PHYSICAL EXAMINATION

Clinical signs of feline asthma are variable with 2 major common clinical presentations. The first is an asthmatic crisis ("status asthmaticus") and the second is the chronic clinical presentation of cough and increased breathing effort. There are gradations in the severity and frequency of clinical signs. Cats in status asthmaticus present with open mouth breathing, tachypnea, and increased abdominal effort ("push") on exhalation. Signs in cats with chronic clinical signs can go unnoticed and untreated by the owner for a long period of time, allowing progression of pathologic changes. It is estimated that 10% to 15% of cats present for vomiting or paroxysmal hacking and coughing[4,7] rather than respiratory distress. Complaints of hacking up hairballs mimicking cough can inadvertently lead to gastrointestinal, not respiratory workups, making identification of a chronic asthmatic patient more challenging.

Classic physical examination findings include cough, expiratory wheeze, and tachypnea.[3–5] Some cats lack abnormalities; however, it is often easy to elicit a cough with gentle tracheal palpation. Aside from these findings, the physical examination is relatively nonspecific, making it important to combine physical examination findings with historical information and results of diagnostic tests to reach a diagnosis of asthma.

DIFFERENTIAL DIAGNOSES

Because there is no single test to diagnose feline asthma definitively, it is important to rule out other diseases that may mimic clinicopathologic features of asthma. Many of these can be relatively easily differentiated using diagnostics such as thoracic radiographs; others warrant more in-depth discussion given their remarkably similar clinical presentations and radiographic findings compared with allergic asthma.

Chronic Bronchitis

Chronic bronchitis is common in cats and shares many clinical features with asthma such as chronic cough. It is thought to arise secondary to a previous airway insult such as respiratory infections or inhaled irritants. A previous airway insult leads to permanent damage to the airways and results in many of the same historical, physical, examination, and radiographic features of asthma. Although cats with either disorder can have a bronchial pattern on thoracic radiographs, cats with asthma have bronchoconstriction in response to inhaled aeroallergen or nonspecific stimulation by inhaled irritants, which results in "air-trapping" that can be visualized on thoracic radiographs as hyperlucent lung fields and displacement of the diaphragm caudally. This should be at least partially reversible with the use of bronchodilators in asthmatic cats. Cats with chronic bronchitis do not have spontaneous bronchoconstriction, although they can have fixed airflow limitation secondary to cellular infiltrates or remodeling changes. Both disorders have differences in cellular infiltrates identified on bronchoalveolar lavage fluid (BALF) cytology with some overlap. Feline allergic asthma is primarily characterized by the presence of eosinophilic inflammation; thus, there should be a predominance ($\geq$17% eosinophils) identified in the BALF.[9] Chronic bronchitis should result in primarily nondegenerate neutrophilic inflammation in BALF. Despite this, there is not always a clear-cut distinction based on BALF as chronic asthma may cause damage to the airways, resulting in some neutrophilic inflammation.[7]

Aelurostrongylosis

Several pulmonary parasitic diseases, including *Aelurostrongylus abstrusus*, can result in similar clinical findings to those seen in asthma, including eosinophilic airway inflammation. *Aelurostrongylus* is a metastrongyloid nematode that infects cats through ingestion of snails, slugs, or paratenic hosts. Radiographically, bronchial to bronchointerstitial lung patterns are typically noted. Although airway eosinophilia is seen with this parasite and with allergic asthma, *Aelurostrongylus* infection can be differentiated by the presence of larvae on BALF cytology or fecal Baermann examination.[10] Because the lack of larvae in these samples does not exclude a diagnosis of *Aelurostrongylus*, empiric treatment with fenbendazole is recommended to more confidently rule out this disorder.

Heartworm Associated Respiratory Disease

Infection with *Dirofilaria immitis* has been proposed to result in heartworm associated respiratory disease (HARD). A preliminary study suggested that death of immature L5 larvae in pulmonary arteries triggers eosinophilic inflammation in the surrounding airways and pulmonary parenchyma.[11] Thus, the presence of adult heartworms might not be necessary for this disease to occur if it is mediated primarily by the larval stage. Diagnostics such as heartworm antigen tests or echocardiography to identify adult heartworms would not not useful in ruling out HARD. HARD should be considered in any cat in an endemic region with appropriate clinicopathologic features and a positive heartworm antibody test that is not receiving heartworm-preventive medication.[12] In addition, there is evidence to suggest that the heartworm endosymbiont, *Wolhbachia*, could contribute to bronchial hyperreactivity in cats with HARD.[13] Thus, it might be useful to treat cats suspected to be affected with HARD with a combination of selamectin to prevent development of larvae beyond the L4 stage as well as doxycycline to eliminate *Wolhbachia.*

Toxocariasis

Toxocara cati infection is relatively common in the pet cat population. Experimentally, pulmonary and transtracheal migration induces pulmonary and vascular disease in affected cats.[14,15] Experimental *T cati* infection also induces bronchointerstitial lesions on thoracic radiographs and causes BALF eosinophilia; however, cats with *T cati* were clinically asymptomatic and did not seem to have airway hyperresponsiveness, a defining feature of asthma.[16] The role of *T cati* as a differential for spontaneous feline asthma is unclear because airway lesions may be incidental; however, this deserves further study.

Infectious Airway Disease

Airway infection or pneumonia in the cat can result in similar presenting complaints and radiographic findings to those of cats with asthma. See Chapter 7 in this edition for further details. (It refers to the chapter "on bacterial pneumonia" by Jonathan Dear).

DIAGNOSTICS

Diagnosis of feline asthma is based on a combination of appropriate clinical signs and physical examination findings as well as diagnostic testing.

Clinicopathologic Findings

In general, clinicopathologic abnormalities of cats with asthma are nonspecific. Complete blood cell counts have revealed peripheral eosinophilia in 17% to 46% of cases,[3–5,7] but this does not correlate with the degree of airway eosinophilia.[4,5,7] There are no specific serum biochemical or urinalysis abnormalities associated with feline asthma.

Thoracic Imaging

Common findings on thoracic radiography in asthmatic cats include a bronchial or bronchointerstitial pattern.[3–7] Collapse of a lung lobe, particularly the right middle lung lobe, presumably secondary to mucus trapping and atelectasis, can also occur in a minority of cats.[3,6] Lack of radiographic abnormalities does not rule out feline asthma because radiographs can be normal in up to 23% of cases.[3] In addition, as mentioned previously, other diseases can result in similar radiographic findings.

Computed tomography (CT) is used in the evaluation of human asthmatic patients.[17–19] Thoracic CT of cats with lower airway disease can identify abnormalities such as bronchial wall thickening, patchy alveolar patterns, and bronchiectasis[20]; however, these findings have not been compared among cats with different forms of lower airway disease. Thoracic CT likely would identify subtle lesions in cats that would not be appreciated on survey radiographs (**Fig. 1**). CT can be performed in cats using a plexiglass chamber allowing acquisition of images without chemical or manual restraint.[21] This provides an important benefit in cats with respiratory distress unable to tolerate the stress of being restrained for radiography. Preliminary studies suggest CT is capable of discriminating differences in lung attenuation and bronchial wall thickening in cats with experimentally induced asthma compared with healthy research cats.[22] Further study is needed to determine the role of thoracic CT in pet cats with asthma.

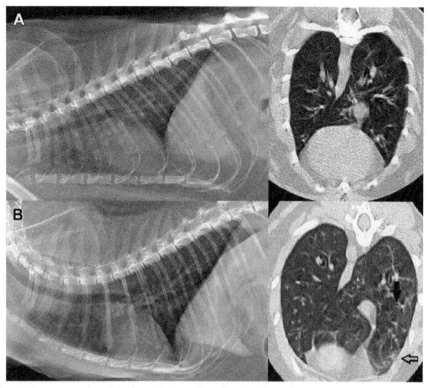

Fig. 1. Representative right lateral thoracic radiographic and computed tomographic (CT) images of 2 awake cats with naturally occurring asthma. CT images were obtained with the cats positioned in a restraining device without the use of anesthetics. The lateral thoracic radiograph of both demonstrates a moderate, diffuse bronchointerstitial lung pattern. On the thoracic CT image of cat (*A*), there is minimal bronchial wall thickening. On the thoracic CT image of cat (*B*), there is prominent bronchial wall thickening (*filled arrow*). In addition, there is a ground-glass appearance to the pulmonary parenchyma particularly in the right lateral lung fields (*open arrow*) with a slight haziness of the lung parenchyma and vasculature from motion artifact. Overall, the CT scan of cat B has increased lung attenuation, whereas cat A has less opaque lung parenchyma despite cat A's lung field being less aerated than cat B, highlighting the benefits of CT compared with thoracic radiography in assessing the severity of structural changes of the airways and pulmonary parenchyma. (*Courtesy of* Isabelle Masseau, DVM, PhD, DACVR, Columbia, MO.)

Bronchoscopy and Bronchoalveolar Lavage Cytology

Bronchoscopy is useful for visual inspection and collection of samples from cats with lower airway disease. Lesions include mucus accumulation, mucosal hyperemia, epithelial irregularities, airway collapse and stenosis, as well as bronchiectasis, although unfortunately, these abnormalities do not discriminate between asthma and other forms of lower respiratory disease.[23] Bronchoalveolar lavage fluid samples for cytologic examination can be collected using bronchoscopy or via a blind technique. Eosinophilic inflammation is noted on BALF cytology of asthmatic cats; however, what constitutes normal cellular percentages in BALF fluid is controversial. Reported "normal" eosinophil percentages in cats have ranged from 0% to 83%.[24–27] In many of these studies, healthy cats have been defined as those free of clinical signs. In human asthmatics, airway inflammation can be present despite the absence of overt symptoms,[28,29] and subclinical inflammation has also been documented in pet cats.[30] Thus, it is possible that some healthy control cats in studies of feline BALF cytology were not appropriate and a cutoff of $\geq$17% BALF eosinophils in pet cats has been proposed as abnormal for some studies.[9,24] Finally, as discussed previously, parasitic diseases result in airway eosinophilia; thus, eosinophilic inflammation is not specific to feline asthma. The findings of eosinophilic airway inflammation should be interpreted in conjunction with clinical signs and diagnostic testing.

Adjunctive Testing

In addition to routine blood testing, thoracic imaging, bronchoscopic examination, and BALF cytology, other diagnostics are used to support a diagnosis of feline asthma and eliminate alternative diagnoses.

Culture of BALF, regardless of whether organisms are detected on cytology, is warranted. In addition, if cultures of *Mycoplasma spp* cannot be performed, PCR should be considered because this is one of the more common opportunistic pathogens in feline lower airway disease.[31] Cats with airway eosinophilia should have a heartworm antibody/antigen test to evaluate for HARD and a fecal floatation and Baermann examination for *T cati* and *A abstrusus*, respectively. It is important to realize that normal results do not rule these diseases out completely.

Allergy Testing

Allergy testing by intradermal skin testing or serum allergen-specific IgE can be used to identify sensitizing allergens implicated in disease, although these are not commonly used in pet cats with asthma. With appropriate identification, allergen avoidance or, in the future, allergen-specific immunotherapy might be used to reduce or eliminate clinical signs in affected cats (see Treatment section).

Pulmonary Function Testing

An important clinical feature of asthma is airflow limitation that is at least partially reversible with bronchodilators. In humans, spirometry is used to gauge lung function. Spirometry requires patient compliance to exhale through a mouthpiece forcefully, making it unsuitable for cats. Alternative pulmonary function testing in cats includes tidal breathing flow-volume loops using a tight fitting face mask, forced expiratory flow-volume curves using a thoracic compression technique, barometric whole body plethysmography (BWBP), and ventilator-acquired lung mechanics.[32–36] Pulmonary function testing is reviewed in chapter 9 of this edition and refers to the chapter by Balakrishnan and Lesley King.

There has been growing interest in using BWBP as a noninvasive test to differentiate between feline asthma and chronic bronchitis. Bronchoprovocation using BWBP discriminates normal cats from cats with lower airway disease,[37] although it is important to understand that BWBP is influenced by the respiratory cycle and does not directly measure airway resistance.[38] Cats with asthma were more likely to demonstrate airflow limitation in response to challenge with an indirect bronchoprovocant than cats with chronic bronchitis.[37] In addition, there was a correlation between the degree and type of airway inflammation and airflow limitation measured by BWBP in spontaneous feline bronchial disease.[39] Namely, cats with airway eosinophilia demonstrated airway hyperresponsiveness at lower doses of the bronchoprovocant than cats with airway neutrophilia. The gold standard technique to measure airway resistance is direct pulmonary mechanics. In experimental feline asthma, ventilator-acquired pulmonary mechanics allow direct and specific calculations of airway resistance and have particular value in assessing effects of therapy on airflow limitation.[22,32,40] Additional studies are needed to determine how well these 2 types of pulmonary function tests correlate.[37,40,41]

TREATMENT

The mainstay of therapy for feline asthma consists of lifelong steroids with or without bronchodilators. Unfortunately, these medications are not effective in all cats, can be associated with adverse effects, and are contraindicated in some cats with concurrent diseases. Therapies that might help to reverse the underlying immunopathology of asthma or could be used as adjuncts in refractory asthma are being investigated in experimental feline asthma models. Although these models are important in identifying therapies that may be effective in asthma, they might not accurately reflect all aspects of spontaneous asthma. Thus, it is critical that studies are repeated in pet cats with asthma.

Traditional Therapies

Glucocorticoids

Steroids are potent anti-inflammatories that have long been used for the treatment of feline asthma. They are most often administered orally in the form of prednisolone; however, inhaled therapy using a spacing chamber (Aerokat; Trudell Medical International, Ontario, Canada) is becoming more commonplace. There are no prospective, controlled studies evaluating the use of glucocorticoids in cats with spontaneous asthma; however, glucocorticoids are considered to be an effective therapy in most cats. Many retrospective studies have reported a beneficial response to glucocorticoids.[3–6] Unfortunately, therapeutic response in these studies is often based on improvement in clinical signs without documenting improvement in airway inflammation or hyperresponsiveness. Given the waxing and waning nature of the clinical signs of asthma, it is difficult to assess the true effectiveness of therapy based on clinical signs alone.

In experimental feline asthma, both oral prednisone (10 mg/d) and inhaled flunisolide (500 μg/d) significantly decreased airway eosinophilia compared with placebo.[42] Using a different experimental feline asthma model, fluticasone propionate with salmeterol (500 μg fluticasone/50 μg salmeterol twice daily) was as effective as oral prednisolone (2 mg/d) at reducing airway inflammation in acute asthma.[43] In a follow-up study by the same group, oral prednisolone (2 mg/d) was compared with inhaled salmeterol (50 μg twice a day) over a 4-day period.[44] Only oral prednisolone was capable of eliminating the late phase asthmatic reaction in response to inhaled allergen.[44] Although an effective dose in pet cats has not been established, comparison of varying doses of inhaled fluticasone (44, 110, or 220 μg twice daily) suggests all are equipotent in controlling airway eosinophilia in experimental asthma.[45]

Bronchodilators

Bronchodilators are critical to reduce bronchoconstriction in acute asthma attacks. However, they should not be used for monotherapy because they fail to control the airway inflammation that exacerbates airway hyperresponsiveness.[8] Several different types of bronchodilators have been assessed, mostly in experimentally asthmatic cats, including methylxanthines,[46,47] short-acting and long-acting β-2 agonists (SABA[5,46,48–50] and LABA,[44,46,48] respectively) and anticholinergics.[46,48,49] When using a compound that directly constricts smooth muscle (ie, carbachol), inhalation of a bronchodilator via a metered dose inhaler and nebulization were equally effective in blunting airway hyperresponsiveness.[48] Also, SABA were more potent than LABA and with combination SABA/anticholinergic bronchodilator therapy, synergism was noted.[48] Interestingly, after specific allergen bronchoprovocation, bronchodilators did not improve time to recovery compared with no treatment.[49] For this reason, the authors prefer use of the injectable bronchodilator terbutaline in pet cats with life-threatening status asthmaticus. Although SABA are critical in treating life-threatening bronchoconstriction, overuse by inhalation has been associated with increased risk of death in human asthmatics.[51] Inhalant albuterol is a racemic mixture consisting of the R-enantiomer, which possesses bronchodilatory properties, and the S-enantiomer (initially thought inert), which promotes bronchospasm and is pro-inflammatory.[52] With repeated use, the S-enantiomer preferentially accumulates in the lung because of slower metabolism/clearance, enhancing bronchoconstrictive and proinflammatory effects.[53] Chronic use (twice daily for 2 weeks) in healthy cats induced de novo neutrophilic airway inflammation; in experimentally asthmatic cats, esoinophilic airway inflammation was exacerbated.[52] This exacerbation indicates that although inhaled albuterol can be an important therapy for acute bronchoconstriction (especially as at-home treatment), it should not be used in the daily management of asthmatic cats. A single isomer form of R-albuterol (levalbuterol) is available, is not associated with negative adverse effects, and could be considered an option for chronic therapy.

Experimental Therapies

Allergen-specific immunotherapy

No therapy to date reverses the underlying immunopathology associated with spontaneous feline allergic asthma. Allergen-specific immunotherapy has emerged as a potentially curative therapy in human medicine as it is proposed to reverse the T helper 2-mediated allergic response by inducing immunologic tolerance to allergen. Several different protocols have been investigated in an experimental model of feline asthma using an abbreviated or "rush" administration (rush immunotherapy, RIT) and have successfully diminished airway eosinophilia.[54–56] Before pet cats with asthma can be treated, allergens implicated in airway sensitization must be identified. Using cats experimentally sensitized to Bermuda grass or house dust mite, the sensitivity and specificity of intradermal skin testing and 2 different forms of serum allergen testing using either an FcεR1α-based ELISA or an enzymoimmunometric assay were investigated.[57] The sensitivity of the IDST was greater than the FcεR1α-based ELISA (ie, better screening test); however, both were specific (ie, suitable for allergen selection for RIT). Disappointingly, the enzymoimmunometric assay produced unreliable results including failure to detect allergen-specific IgE and identification of allergens to which the cats had not been sensitized. Future studies should be performed to evaluate more rigorously the accuracy of diagnostic laboratories offering allergen-specific IgE testing. To determine the importance of closely matched allergens for use in RIT, an additional study was performed in experimentally asthmatic cats.[58] Use of allergens not implicated in sensitization or use of only 1 of 2 sensitizing allergens in RIT still led to reductions in airway eosinophilia. However, only closely matched allergens had the potential to induce an immunologic cure by induction of tolerance, which could potentially allow discontinuation of therapy with permanent benefit.

Omega-3 fatty acids/neutraceuticals

Omega-3 Polyunsaturated fatty acids are anti-inflammatory due to reduction of arachadonic acid in cell membranes available for production of inflammatory eicosanoids.[59] The use of dietary ω-3 polyunsaturated fatty acids in combination with the antioxidant, luteolin, has been evaluated in experimental feline asthma.[60] This treatment failed to resolve airway eosinophilia, but diminished airway hyperresponsiveness as assessed by BWBP. Although clearly unsuitable as monotherapy, additional studies in pet cats with asthma might help determine if they could be used as adjunctive therapy.

Inhaled lidocaine
Lidocaine has received interest in human medicine as a potential treatment of severe asthma[61–63] and has been investigated in an experimental feline asthma model.[64] In the latter study, nebulized lidocaine (2 mg/kg q8h) was administered to healthy and experimentally asthmatic cats for 2 weeks. Lidocaine decreased airway hyperresponsiveness without decreasing airway eosinophilia. Importantly, no adverse effects were noted in the cats despite the known sensitivity of cats to injectable lidocaine. Further study is needed to determine if lidocaine might be useful to treat airflow limitation in spontaneous feline asthma.

Tyrosine kinase inhibitors
Blockade of key cell signaling pathways involved in the immunopathogenesis of asthma could lead to novel avenues of treatment. Both receptor and nonreceptor tyrosine kinase inhibitors (TKIs) have potential in this regard. For example, stem cell factor, the growth factor for the c-kit receptor, is associated with proliferation and activation of both mast cells and eosinophils[65] and, in experimental feline asthma, these can be inhibited with TKIs such as masitinib.[32] Cats receiving masitinib (50 mg/d by mouth) showed decreases in BALF eosinophilia and lung compliance as measured by ventilator-acquired pulmonary mechanics. Unfortunately, side effects were dose-limiting. Inhibition of the janus kinase cytokine signaling pathway by a nonreceptor TKI was also evaluated in feline asthma.[66] In a preliminary study, cats showed reduction of airway eosinophilia without a significant effect on airway hyperresponsiveness.

Stem cells
Stem cells have been studied for the treatment of a variety of respiratory disorders including asthma. Murine asthma models have demonstrated that stem cells can reduce airway eosinophilia, airway hyperresponsiveness, and airway remodeling.[67–70] Early data suggest that the most beneficial effects of intravenously administered allogeneic feline adipose-derived stem cells in experimental asthma might be amelioration of airway remodeling as assessed by thoracic CT scans.[71] These stem cells are not the same as commercially available products, and further studies are needed before stem cells are recommended for feline asthma.

Ineffective Therapies

Leukotriene antagonists are part of the arsenal of medications used for treatment of human asthmatics. Unfortunately cysteinyl leukotrienes do not seem to be important mediators of feline asthma[72,73] and a clinical trial with the leukotriene antagonist, zafirlukast, failed to reduce airway eosinophilia or hyperresponsiveness in experimental feline asthma.[42] Serotonin is a preformed mediator in mast cells and is thought to be important in mediating bronchoconstriction in response to allergen exposure.[73,74] Cyproheptadine, a nonspecific serotonin antagonist, at a low dose (2 mg q12h by mouth) failed to significantly reduce airway reactivity and airway inflammation in experimentally asthmatic cats.[42] A subsequent study[75] evaluated a higher dose of cyproheptadine (8 mg q12h by mouth) based on a pharmacokinetic study, suggesting cats may require substantially higher doses than what has been traditionally recommended to reach therapeutic concentrations.[76] Even at this dose, cyproheptadine was ineffective at reducing airway eosinophilia. Because hyperresponsiveness was not evaluated in this study, it is uncertain if the higher dose could alleviate airflow limitation. Although not advocated for monotherapy, the higher dose deserves further study to evaluate its bronchodilatory properties. Histamine, like serotonin, is present in the granules of mast cells and could have similar effects on airway reactivity.[74,77–80] A study investigating the second-generation antihistamine, cetirizine (5 mg q12h by mouth), found that airway eosinophilia was not significantly diminished.[75] The effect of cetirizine on airway hyperresponsiveness is currently not known and further study is needed before this therapy can be recommended.

A salivary tripeptide (feG-COOH) identified as a modulator of the immune response reduced allergen-induced airway inflammation in other animal models of asthma.[81,82] Chronic administration of feG-COOH (1 mg/kg/d for 2 wk) did not blunt airway eosinophilia compared with placebo in experimental feline asthma and cannot be advocated.[83] Oral doxycycline (5 mg/kg twice daily) failed to blunt airway eosinophilia or hyperresponsiveness.[44] N-acetylcysteine is a mucolytic with antioxidant properties that could have a benefit in asthma; however, nebulized delivery in humans is known to induce bronchospasm. Similarly, in experimentally asthmatic cats, nebulization of N-acetylcysteine increased baseline airway resistance by an average of approximately 150% and should not be administered by this route.[40]

MONITORING

Traditionally, titration of therapy in asthmatic cats relies on observation of reduction in clinical signs. However, clinical signs of asthma can wax and wane, making it difficult to determine if the reduction in clinical signs is related to a true effect of the medication. Recently, a retrospective study investigated the presence of inflammation on BALF cytology after initial treatment with high-dose glucocorticoids and found that despite cats having no clinical signs of asthma at the time of sampling, many had subclinical inflammation noted on BALF cytology.[30] Importantly, unchecked airway inflammation can lead to irreversible remodeling resulting in a decline in lung function.[84–86] Until a less invasive diagnostic test is developed, repeated analysis of BALF cytology could be necessary before making alterations in treatment protocols in asthmatic cats.

SUMMARY

Much work must be done to define feline asthma better and discriminate it from other lower airway diseases. Importantly, accurately identifying asthmatics will help more appropriately select candidates for targeted therapies acting along the allergic cascade. Although many experimental therapies are being investigated in feline asthma, work is still needed to determine if these will be beneficial in our pet cat population.

REFERENCES

1. Reinero CR. Advances in the understanding of pathogenesis, and diagnostics and therapeutics for feline allergic asthma. Vet J 2011;190(1):28–33.
2. Padrid P. Chronic bronchitis and asthma in cats. In: Bonagura J, Twedt D, editors. Current veterinary therapy XIV. Philadelphia: WB Saunders; 2009. p. 650–8.
3. Adamama-Moraitou KK, Patsikas MN, Koutinas AF. Feline lower airway disease: a retrospective study of 22 naturally occurring cases from Greece. J Feline Med Surg 2004;6(4):227–33.
4. Corcoran BM, Foster DJ, Fuentes VL. Feline asthma syndrome: a retrospective study of the clinical presentation in 29 cats. J Small Anim Pract 1995;36(11): 481–8.

5. Dye JA, McKiernan BC, Rozanski EA, et al. Bronchopulmonary disease in the cat: historical, physical, radiographic, clinicopathologic, and pulmonary functional evaluation of 24 affected and 15 healthy cats. J Vet Intern Med 1996; 10(6):385–400.
6. Foster SF, Allan GS, Martin P, et al. Twenty-five cases of feline bronchial disease (1995-2000). J Feline Med Surg 2004;6(3):181–8.
7. Moise NS, Wiedenkeller D, Yeager AE, et al. Clinical, radiographic, and bronchial cytologic features of cats with bronchial disease: 65 cases (1980-1986). J Am Vet Med Assoc 1989;194(10):1467–73.
8. Busse W, Camargo C Jr, Boushey H, et al. Expert panel report 3: guidelines for the diagnosis and management of asthma. 2007. Available at: http://www.nhlbi. nih.gov/guidelines/asthma/asthgdln.htm. Accessed June 24, 2013.
9. Nafe LA, DeClue AE, Lee-Fowler TM, et al. Evaluation of biomarkers in bronchoalveolar lavage fluid for discrimination between asthma and chronic bronchitis in cats. Am J Vet Res 2010;71(5):583–91.
10. Lacorcia L, Gasser RB, Anderson GA, et al. Comparison of bronchoalveolar lavage fluid examination and other diagnostic techniques with the Baermann technique for detection of naturally occurring Aelurostrongylus abstrusus infection in cats. J Am Vet Med Assoc 2009;235(1):43–9.
11. Dillon AR, Blagburn B, Tillson D, et al. Immature heartworm infection produces pulmonary parenchymal, airway, and vascular disease in cats [abstract]. J Vet Intern Med 2007;21(3):608–9.
12. Lee AC, Atkins CE. Understanding feline heartworm infection: disease, diagnosis, and treatment. Top Companion Anim Med 2010;25(4):224–30.
13. Garcia-Guasch L, Caro-Vadillo A, Manubens-Grau J, et al. Is Wolbachia participating in the bronchial reactivity of cats with heartworm associated respiratory disease? Vet Parasitol 2013;196(1–2):130–5.
14. Sprent JF. The life history and development of Toxocara cati (Schrank 1788) in the domestic cat. Parasitology 1956;46(1–2):54–78.
15. Swerczek TW, Nielsen SW, Helmboldt CF. Ascariasis causing pulmonary arterial hyperplasia in cats. Res Vet Sci 1970;11(1):103–4.
16. Dillon AR, Tillson DM, Hathcock J, et al. Lung histopathology, radiography, high-resolution computed tomography, and bronchio-alveolar lavage cytology are altered by Toxocara cati infection in cats and is independent of development of adult intestinal parasites. Vet Parasitol 2013;193(4):413–26.
17. Niimi A, Matsumoto H, Amitani R, et al. Airway wall thickness in asthma assessed by computed tomography. Relation to clinical indices. Am J Respir Crit Care Med 2000;162(4 Pt 1):1518–23.
18. Niimi A, Matsumoto H, Takemura M, et al. Clinical assessment of airway remodeling in asthma: utility of computed tomography. Clin Rev Allergy Immunol 2004; 27(1):45–58.
19. Mitsunobu F, Tanizaki Y. The use of computed tomography to assess asthma severity. Curr Opin Allergy Clin Immunol 2005;5(1):85–90.
20. Oliveira CR, Mitchell MA, O'Brien RT. Thoracic computed tomography in feline patients without use of chemical restraint. Vet Radiol Ultrasound 2011;52(4): 368–76.
21. Oliveira CR, Ranallo FN, Pijanowski GJ, et al. The VetMousetrap: a device for computed tomographic imaging of the thorax of awake cats. Vet Radiol Ultrasound 2011;52(1):41–52.
22. Masseau I, Chang C, LeFloch M, et al. Assessment of airway hyperresponsiveness in tandem with remodeling using pulmonary mechanics and computed

tomography in experimental feline asthma [abstract R-3]. J Vet Intern Med 2013; 27(3):754.

23. Johnson LR, Vernau W. Bronchoscopic findings in 48 cats with spontaneous lower respiratory tract disease (2002-2009). J Vet Intern Med 2011;25(2):236–43.

24. Hawkins EC, DeNicola DB, Kuehn NF. Bronchoalveolar lavage in the evaluation of pulmonary disease in the dog and cat. State of the art. J Vet Intern Med 1990; 4(5):267–74.

25. McCarthy GM, Quinn PJ. Bronchoalveolar lavage in the cat: cytological findings. Can J Vet Res 1989;53(3):259–63.

26. McCarthy GM, Quinn PJ. Age-related changes in protein concentrations in serum and respiratory tract lavage fluid obtained from cats. Am J Vet Res 1991;52(2):254–60.

27. Padrid PA, Feldman BF, Funk K, et al. Cytologic, microbiologic, and biochemical analysis of bronchoalveolar lavage fluid obtained from 24 healthy cats. Am J Vet Res 1991;52(8):1300–7.

28. Laprise C, Laviolette M, Boutet M, et al. Asymptomatic airway hyperresponsiveness: relationships with airway inflammation and remodelling. Eur Respir J 1999; 14(1):63–73.

29. Obase Y, Shimoda T, Kawano T, et al. Bronchial hyperresponsiveness and airway inflammation in adolescents with asymptomatic childhood asthma. Allergy 2003;58(3):213–20.

30. Cocayne CG, Reinero CR, DeClue AE. Subclinical airway inflammation despite high-dose oral corticosteroid therapy in cats with lower airway disease. J Feline Med Surg 2011;13(8):558–63.

31. Foster SF, Martin P, Braddock JA, et al. A retrospective analysis of feline bronchoalveolar lavage cytology and microbiology (1995-2000). J Feline Med Surg 2004;6(3):189–98.

32. Lee-Fowler TM, Guntur V, Dodam J, et al. The tyrosine kinase inhibitor masitinib blunts airway inflammation and improves associated lung mechanics in a feline model of chronic allergic asthma. Int Arch Allergy Immunol 2012;158(4):369–74.

33. Bark H, Epstein A, Bar-Yishay E, et al. Non-invasive forced expiratory flow-volume curves to measure lung function in cats. Respir Physiol Neurobiol 2007;155(1): 49–54.

34. Hoffman AM, Dhupa N, Cimetti L. Airway reactivity measured by barometric whole-body plethysmography in healthy cats. Am J Vet Res 1999;60(12):1487–92.

35. Kirschvink N, Leemans J, Delvaux F, et al. Non-invasive assessment of airway responsiveness in healthy and allergen-sensitised cats by use of barometric whole body plethysmography. Vet J 2007;173(2):343–52.

36. McKiernan BC, Johnson LR. Clinical pulmonary function testing in dogs and cats. Vet Clin North Am Small Anim Pract 1992;22(5):1087–99.

37. Hirt RA, Galler A, Shibly S, et al. Airway hyperresponsiveness to adenosine 5'-monophosphate in feline chronic inflammatory lower airway disease. Vet J 2011;187(1):54–9.

38. Bates J, Irvin C, Brusasco V, et al. The use and misuse of Penh in animal models of lung disease. Am J Respir Cell Mol Biol 2004;31(3):373–4.

39. Allerton FJ, Leemans J, Tual C, et al. Correlation of bronchoalveolar eosinophilic percentage with airway responsiveness in cats with chronic bronchial disease. J Small Anim Pract 2013;54(5):258–64.

40. Reinero CR, Lee-Fowler TM, Dodam JR, et al. Endotracheal nebulization of N-acetylcysteine increases airway resistance in cats with experimental asthma. J Feline Med Surg 2011;13(2):69–73.

41. Chang CH, Dodam JR, Cohn LA, et al. Validation of direct and indirect bronchoprovocation testing using ventilator-acquired pulmonary mechanics in healthy and experimentally asthmatic cats [abstract R-5]. J Vet Intern Med 2013;27(3):753.
42. Reinero CR, Decile KC, Byerly JR, et al. Effects of drug treatment on inflammation and hyperreactivity of airways and on immune variables in cats with experimentally induced asthma. Am J Vet Res 2005;66(7):1121–7.
43. Leemans J, Kirschvink N, Clercx C, et al. Effect of short-term oral and inhaled corticosteroids on airway inflammation and responsiveness in a feline acute asthma model. Vet J 2012;192(1):41–8.
44. Leemans J, Kirschvink N, Bernaerts F, et al. Salmeterol or doxycycline do not inhibit acute bronchospasm and airway inflammation in cats with experimentally-induced asthma. Vet J 2012;192(1):49–56.
45. Cohn LA, DeClue AE, Cohen RL, et al. Effects of fluticasone propionate dosage in an experimental model of feline asthma. J Feline Med Surg 2010;12(2):91–6.
46. Leemans J, Kirschvink N, Gustin P. A comparison of in vitro relaxant responses to ipratropium bromide, beta-adrenoceptor agonists and theophylline in feline bronchial smooth muscle. Vet J 2012;193(1):228–33.
47. Stursberg U, Zenker I, Hecht S, et al. Use of propentofylline in feline bronchial disease: prospective, randomized, positive-controlled study. J Am Anim Hosp Assoc 2010;46(5):318–26.
48. Leemans J, Kirschvink N, Bernaerts F, et al. A pilot study comparing the antispasmodic effects of inhaled salmeterol, salbutamol and ipratropium bromide using different aerosol devices on muscarinic bronchoconstriction in healthy cats. Vet J 2009;180(2):236–45.
49. Leemans J, Kirschvink N, Clercx C, et al. Functional response to inhaled salbutamol and/or ipratropium bromide in Ascaris suum-sensitised cats with allergen-induced bronchospasms. Vet J 2010;186(1):76–83.
50. Rozanski EA, Hoffman AM. Pulmonary function testing in small animals. Clin Tech Small Anim Pract 1999;14(4):237–41.
51. Spitzer WO, Suissa S, Ernst P, et al. The use of beta-agonists and the risk of death and near death from asthma. N Engl J Med 1992;326(8):501–6.
52. Reinero CR, Delgado C, Spinka C, et al. Enantiomer-specific effects of albuterol on airway inflammation in healthy and asthmatic cats. Int Arch Allergy Immunol 2009;150(1):43–50.
53. Dhand R, Goode M, Reid R, et al. Preferential pulmonary retention of (S)-albuterol after inhalation of racemic albuterol. Am J Respir Crit Care Med 1999;160(4):1136–41.
54. Lee-Fowler TM, Cohn LA, DeClue AE, et al. Evaluation of subcutaneous versus mucosal (intranasal) allergen-specific rush immunotherapy in experimental feline asthma. Vet Immunol Immunopathol 2009;129(1–2):49–56.
55. Reinero CR, Byerly JR, Berghaus RD, et al. Rush immunotherapy in an experimental model of feline allergic asthma. Vet Immunol Immunopathol 2006;110(1–2):141–53.
56. Reinero CR, Cohn LA, Delgado C, et al. Adjuvanted rush immunotherapy using CpG oligodeoxynucleotides in experimental feline allergic asthma. Vet Immunol Immunopathol 2008;121(3–4):241–50.
57. Lee-Fowler TM, Cohn LA, DeClue AE, et al. Comparison of intradermal skin testing (IDST) and serum allergen-specific IgE determination in an experimental model of feline asthma. Vet Immunol Immunopathol 2009;132(1):46–52.
58. Reinero C, Lee-Fowler T, Chang CH, et al. Beneficial cross-protection of allergen-specific immunotherapy on airway eosinophilia using unrelated or a

partial repertoire of allergen(s) implicated in experimental feline asthma. Vet J 2012;192(3):412–6.

59. Calder PC. Polyunsaturated fatty acids and inflammation. Prostaglandins Leukot Essent Fatty Acids 2006;75(3):197–202.

60. Leemans J, Cambier C, Chandler T, et al. Prophylactic effects of omega-3 poly-unsaturated fatty acids and luteolin on airway hyperresponsiveness and inflam-mation in cats with experimentally-induced asthma. Vet J 2010;184(1):111–4.

61. Decco ML, Neeno TA, Hunt LW, et al. Nebulized lidocaine in the treatment of severe asthma in children: a pilot study. Ann Allergy Asthma Immunol 1999; 82(1):29–32.

62. Hunt LW, Frigas E, Butterfield JH, et al. Treatment of asthma with nebulized lido-caine: a randomized, placebo-controlled study. J Allergy Clin Immunol 2004; 113(5):853–9.

63. Hunt LW, Swedlund HA, Gleich GJ. Effect of nebulized lidocaine on severe glucocorticoid-dependent asthma. Mayo Clin Proc 1996;71(4):361–8.

64. Nafe LA, Guntur VP, Dodam JR, et al. Nebulized lidocaine blunts airway hyper-responsiveness in experimental feline asthma. J Feline Med Surg 2013;15(8): 712–6.

65. Guntur VP, Reinero CR. The potential use of tyrosine kinase inhibitors in severe asthma. Curr Opin Allergy Clin Immunol 2012;12(1):68–75.

66. Chang CH, Dodam JR, Cohn LA, et al. An experimental janus kinase (JAK) inhibitor suppressess eosinophilic airway inflammation in feline asthma. In: ACVIM Forum Proceedings. 2013. Available at: http://www.vin.com/Members/ Proceedings/Proceedings.plx?CID=ACVIM2013&Category=&PID=89227&O= Generic. Accessed June 24, 2013.

67. Bonfield TL, Koloze M, Lennon DP, et al. Human mesenchymal stem cells sup-press chronic airway inflammation in the murine ovalbumin asthma model. Am J Physiol Lung Cell Mol Physiol 2010;299(6):L760–70.

68. Firinci F, Karaman M, Baran Y, et al. Mesenchymal stem cells ameliorate the histopathological changes in a murine model of chronic asthma. Int Immuno-pharmacol 2011;11(8):1120–6.

69. Goodwin M, Sueblinvong V, Eisenhauer P, et al. Bone marrow-derived mesen-chymal stromal cells inhibit Th2-mediated allergic airways inflammation in mice. Stem Cells 2011;29(7):1137–48.

70. Ou-Yang HF, Huang Y, Hu XB, et al. Suppression of allergic airway inflammation in a mouse model of asthma by exogenous mesenchymal stem cells. Exp Biol Med (Maywood) 2011;236(12):1461–7.

71. Masseau I, Trzil JE, Chang CH, et al. Stem cell therapy blunts computed tomographic measures of airway remodeling in experimental feline asthma. In: ACVIM Forum Proceedings. 2013. Available at: http://www.vin.com/Members/ Proceedings/Proceedings.plx?CID=ACVIM2013&Category=&PID=89242&O= Generic. Accessed June 24, 2013.

72. Norris CR, Decile KC, Berghaus LJ, et al. Concentrations of cysteinyl leukotri-enes in urine and bronchoalveolar lavage fluid of cats with experimentally induced asthma. Am J Vet Res 2003;64(11):1449–53.

73. Padrid PA, Mitchell RW, Ndukwu IM, et al. Cyproheptadine-induced attenuation of type-I immediate-hypersensitivity reactions of airway smooth muscle from immune-sensitized cats. Am J Vet Res 1995;56(1):109–15.

74. Mitchell RW, Cozzi P, Ndukwu IM, et al. Differential effects of cyclosporine A after acute antigen challenge in sensitized cats in vivo and ex vivo. Br J Pharmacol 1998;123(6):1198–204.

75. Schooley EK, McGee Turner JB, Jiji RD, et al. Effects of cyproheptadine and ce-tirizine on eosinophilic airway inflammation in cats with experimentally induced asthma. Am J Vet Res 2007;68(11):1265–71.
76. Norris CR, Boothe DM, Esparza T, et al. Disposition of cyproheptadine in cats after intravenous or oral administration of a single dose. Am J Vet Res 1998; 59(1):79–81.
77. Banovcin P, Visnovsky P, Korpas J. Pharmacological analysis of reactivity changes in airways due to acute inflammation in cats. Acta Physiol Hung 1987;70(2–3):181–7.
78. Barnes PJ. Histamine and serotonin. Pulm Pharmacol Ther 2001;14(5):329–39.
79. Wenzel SE, Fowler AA 3rd, Schwartz LB. Activation of pulmonary mast cells by bronchoalveolar allergen challenge. In vivo release of histamine and tryptase in atopic subjects with and without asthma. Am Rev Respir Dis 1988;137(5): 1002–8.
80. Wilson AM. The role of antihistamines in asthma management. Treat Respir Med 2006;5(3):149–58.
81. Dery RE, Ulanova M, Puttagunta L, et al. Frontline: inhibition of allergen-induced pulmonary inflammation by the tripeptide feG: a mimetic of a neuro-endocrine pathway. Eur J Immunol 2004;34(12):3315–25.
82. Dery RE, Mathison R, Davison J, et al. Inhibition of allergic inflammation by C-terminal peptides of the prohormone submandibular rat 1 (SMR-1). Int Arch Allergy Immunol 2001;124(1–3):201–4.
83. Eberhardt JM, DeClue AE, Reinero CR. Chronic use of the immunomodulating tripeptide feG-COOH in experimental feline asthma. Vet Immunol Immunopathol 2009;132(2–4):175–80.
84. Norris Reinero CR, Decile KC, Berghaus RD, et al. An experimental model of allergic asthma in cats sensitized to house dust mite or bermuda grass allergen. Int Arch Allergy Immunol 2004;135(2):117–31.
85. Padrid P. Feline asthma. Diagnosis and treatment. Vet Clin North Am Small Anim Pract 2000;30(6):1279–93.
86. Padrid P, Snook S, Finucane T, et al. Persistent airway hyperresponsiveness and histologic alterations after chronic antigen challenge in cats. Am J Respir Crit Care Med 1995;151(1):184–93.

Canine Chronic Bronchitis

Elizabeth Rozanski, DVM

KEYWORDS

- Cough • Inflammatory • Pulmonary pharmacology • Cough suppressant
- Chronic bronchitis

KEY POINTS

- Chronic cough is a syndrome not a final diagnosis.
- Evaluation of potential underlying causes is important to exclude more treatable and curable diseases.
- Chronic bronchitis is an inflammatory disease, and glucocorticoids tapered to the lowest possible dose to control signs are most commonly required.

Canine chronic bronchitis (CCB) is an inflammatory chronic pulmonary disease that results in cough and can lead to exercise intolerance and respiratory distress. Clinical signs vary from mild to severe, with the most severe cases resulting in respiratory failure. The goals of this article are to (1) review an overall approach to diagnosis and management of chronic bronchitis, (2) review pathophysiology associated with chronic bronchitis, and (3) highlight emerging areas and concepts.

OVERVIEW

Cough is defined as a sudden noisy expulsion of air, associated with efforts to clear the airway. Both acute and chronic cough are common presenting complaints for dogs in small animal practice. Other airway sounds may be confused with cough, such as reverse sneezing or temporary airway occlusion from pulling on leash. Additionally, upper airway sounds, such as stridor or stertor, may be confused with cough. As smartphone use becomes more widespread, video recording of cough or other odd respiratory sounds is helpful to clinicians in distinguishing and characterizing cough, especially if sounds are transient or hard to reproduce.

In some dogs, particularly small breed dogs, cough is accepted as normal by many clients, and further evaluation is not pursued until signs are advanced. Inquiry as to the frequency of cough is advised in all dogs because early treatment of airway disease and control of obesity (if indicated) are likely associated with a better outcome than waiting until cough is intractable.

Section of Critical Care, Tufts Cummings School of Veterinary Medicine, 200 Westboro Road, North Grafton, MA 01536, USA
E-mail address: elizabeth.rozanski@tufts.edu

Vet Clin Small Anim 44 (2014) 107–116
http://dx.doi.org/10.1016/j.cvsm.2013.09.005
0195-5616/14/$ – see front matter © 2014 Elsevier Inc. All rights reserved.

There are many possible causes for cough and identification of and therapy for the specific cause of cough is more likely to result in an amelioration of clinical signs than simple supportive care. CCB is defined as cough on most days of the preceding 2 months, without any other cause identified. Therefore, it is important to exclude other causes of cough prior to making a diagnosis of chronic bronchitis. Chronic bronchitis can also coexist with other cardiopulmonary conditions, such as mitral regurgitation or airway collapse, or it can lead to pulmonary hypertension (cor pulmonale) as it progresses.

Common causes of cough in dogs include infectious diseases as well as lung tumors, pleural effusion, upper airway dysfunction with gastroesophageal reflux, interstitial lung disease, and congestive heart failure. Disease due to the canine infectious respiratory disease complex involves *Bordetella bronchiseptica* infection most frequently, but *Mycoplasma* and canine influenza virus are among other infecting organisms.[1] Although infectious disease is most common in puppies and in dogs exposed to other dogs through activities, such as boarding or grooming, it is also a common cause of an exacerbation of signs in older dogs with preexisting cardiopulmonary disease. Dogs that have decompensated after a period of stability should be evaluated for infection.

Lung tumors are often bronchial adenocarcinomas, and, as such, they grow around a bronchus. Mucus and debris can drain into the airway lumen and cause cough. Pleural effusion is a less common cause of cough but is thought to cause cough by diaphragmatic irritation or because of airway compression associated with lung collapse. Upper airway dysfunction (eg, laryngeal paralysis) causes cough by intermittent aspiration of food and liquids. In geriatric dogs, laryngeal paralysis can be associated with pharyngeal dysfunction, which also leads to cough.[2] A recent report described reversible laryngeal dysfunction associated with gastroesophageal reflux in a Saint Bernard dog.[3] This has not been widely appreciated in veterinary medicine, although in people, gastroesophageal reflex disease is a common cause of cough.[4] In brachycephalic dogs, there has been a relationship observed between gastrointestinal and respiratory signs.[5]

Interstitial lung disease more often causes tachypnea and exercise intolerance, although cough is present in some dogs. Congestive heart failure is expected to result in tachypnea and increased respiratory rate at rest before the development of cough, although dogs with heart failure can display a dry cough. Cough has classically been associated with marked left atrial enlargement causing compression of the mainstem bronchi, but a recent study suggested that these dogs likely have airway disease.[6] Tracheal and airway collapse are commonly associated with cough. See the article "Tracheal and Airway Collapse" by Dr Della Maggiore elsewhere in this issue.

CLINICAL APPROACH

Evaluation of dogs with cough starts with review of the recent history and environmental exposures and a complete physical examination. Signalment is helpful in establishing a suspicion of chronic bronchitis, because it is most common in older small breed dogs. Cocker spaniels have been identified with an increased risk of bronchiectasis,[7] which occurs as a sequela to poorly controlled bronchitis in some cases. Pertinent historical considerations include exposure, even if limited, to other dogs/ puppies where infectious disease could be a consideration and evidence of systemic disease, such as exercise intolerance. Exposure to passive (second-hand) smoking or excessive environmental odors/perfumes anecdotally seems to contribute to cough although this has not been scientifically established.[8] Additionally, the nature of cough should be explored, including dry or productive, paroxysmal, constant, or intermittent, and its relation to eating and activity. Voice change or reluctance to bark can support an upper airway disease, such as laryngeal paralysis or hemiparalysis, and indicates that microaspiration should be considered as a cause of cough. Prior use of prescription or home remedies and the perceived effect on the cough should be explored.

A complete physical examination should focus on the cardiopulmonary system as well as identifying signs of systemic disease, including recent weight loss or gain, loss of appetite, and weakness or lethargy. Auscultation of the lungs can provide clues of lower airway disease, although a variety of findings should be anticipated ranging from normal to harsh lung sounds, crackles, or expiratory wheezes. The presence or absence of a murmur should be noted although even when a mitral murmur is detected, chronic cough is more likely of pulmonary rather than cardiac origin. A respiratory arrhythmia is a common auscultatory finding in dogs with chronic bronchitis, thought associated with elevated vagal tone. A cough often is induced by palpation of the trachea; this is useful to better characterize the cough and to exclude other conditions that could be mistaken for cough, such as reverse sneezing. Most dogs with chronic bronchitis are systemically well geriatric dogs, with only persistent productive cough as the major complaint.

Some dogs have syncope associated with cough, or the so-called cough-drop syndrome, which is most likely associated with high vagal tone. A second consideration for dogs with syncope is the presence of pulmonary hypertension, which can occur secondary to chronic tracheobronchial disease.

Diagnostic testing should be tailored to individual patients; however, tests typically performed include baseline laboratory testing, such as a complete blood cell count, chemistry profile, and urinalysis. These laboratory tests are useful in establishing general health and are anticipated to be largely normal in dogs with chronic bronchitis. Peripheral eosinophilia is of particular interest in baseline laboratory results, because circulating eosinophilia can be associated with pulmonary eosinophilia or parasite infection. Other laboratory testing that should be considered includes heartworm antigen testing, fecal analysis for both eggs and lungworm larva, and evaluation of N-terminal prohormone (NT) of pro–brain natriuretic peptide (BNP), a biomarker that is elevated in the presence of left atrial enlargement/congestive heart failure as well as in pulmonary hypertension. Elevated NT pro-BNP should prompt further evaluation by echocardiography.[9]

Lung Function Testing

Pulmonary function testing is widely used in human medicine to better characterize the specific defects in airflow associated with chronic bronchitis. Lung function, although difficult to routinely evaluate in clinical veterinary cases, is markedly affected by chronic bronchitis. As a review, lung function is a combination of (1) adequate gas exchange, which is evaluated by arterial blood gas analysis, pulse oximetry, or end-tidal CO_2 analysis, and (2) work of breathing, as indicated by lung mechanics. Lung mechanics are mathematical descriptions of the relationships between gas flow rates, air volume/tidal volume, and airway pressure changes during breathing. See the article "Updates on Pulmonary Function Testing" by Drs Balakrishnan and King elsewhere in this issue.

In chronic bronchitis, airway lumen narrowing develops from a combination of airway thickening and excessive mucus production and accumulation, which result in increased airway resistance. This is especially pronounced in expiration. Additionally, there may be expiratory flow limitation due to airway collapse and narrowing, which leads to air trapping or dynamic hyperinflation. Hyperinflation subsequently increases the work of breathing and perpetuate lung dysfunction. Importantly, in contrast to asthmatic people, cats, and horses, dogs have little to no naturally occurring bronchoconstriction.

Although pulmonary function testing is simple to perform in dogs, lack of readily available standardized equipment limits its utility at this time. Additionally, subtle deficits in people are most effectively revealed with tests designed to evaluate maximal effort, such as the forced expiratory volume in the first second of expiration, and these are impossible to perform in patients that lack voluntary cooperation. Tidal breathing flow-volume loops have been described in dogs with CCB and demonstrate expiratory flow abnormalities.[10] More practically, two forms of pulmonary function testing are used in dogs, specifically, collection of arterial blood gas samples and use of the 6-minute walk test (6MWT). Arterial blood gas analysis can document mild hypoxemia or an increased alveolar-arterial gradient to support pulmonary dysfunction. The 6MWT is performed by measuring the distance that a dog walks in 6 minutes. Distances of less than 400 m are supportive of significant lung disease.[11] This type of testing could be used to assess dysfunction associated with disease and potentially to monitor therapeutic response to various interventions.

Diagnostic Imaging

Chest radiographs are helpful in evaluating dogs with cough. If diagnostic testing is limited for an individual patient, chest radiographs are the most useful test. Chest radiographs should be evaluated for evidence of bronchial thickening and increased donuts and tramlines (**Fig. 1**). Additional signs consistent with chronic bronchitis include obesity, bronchiectasis, and, less commonly, hyperinflation. Chest radiographs are also useful to exclude other conditions that cause cough, such as congestive heart failure, lung masses, pleural effusion, and interstitial lung disease.

Fluoroscopy is useful for evaluating the tracheal and larger airway for collapse. Ultrasound is useful if an isolated peripheral lesion is found on radiographs or in the presence of pleural effusion but is not useful in bronchitis.

CT, which is widely used in people with airway diseases, is growing in popularity for identification of canine bronchial disease as well. CT scanning usually requires brief general anesthesia, so is commonly combined with evaluation of laryngeal function,

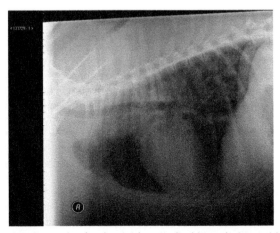

Fig. 1. Right lateral radiograph of a dog with a marked bronchointerstitial pattern consistent with chronic bronchitis.

bronchoscopy, and collection of airway cytology samples in dogs suspected of having CCB. The airway detail shown by CT scanning is much improved compared with routine thoracic radiographs.

Bronchoscopy, if available, is the preferred technique to evaluate and visualize the airway (**Fig. 2**). In a study of chronic bronchitis, all dogs demonstrated irregular mucosal surfaces with a loss of the glistening appearance seen in healthy airways. Often the mucosa was noted as thickened and granular with a roughened appearance. Most dogs in the same study had hyperemia of mucosal vessels and showed partial collapse of bronchi during volume expiration. The presence of excessive mucus in the airways is also consistent with CB.[10,12] In people, bronchoscopy is not required for the diagnosis of chronic bronchitis, with more focus on lung function testing. It is the author's opinion, however, that bronchoscopy provides useful information in dogs with chronic bronchitis and should be pursed if practical.

Airway Sampling

Collection of airway samples for cytology and bacterial culture is useful in further characterizing chronic bronchitis and excluding other causes of cough. Cytology samples are collected by tracheal wash, by blind bronchoalveolar lavage, or with a bronchoscope.[13] The technique chosen reflects clinician preference and the availability of supplies and equipment.

Airway samples for cytologic assessment should be placed in EDTA-containing tubes or submitted in syringes or suction traps. They should be processed promptly to avoid changes in the cell counts and appearance. If analysis is delayed, a small aliquot of the sample should be centrifuged and a direct smear made of the pellet. Respiratory cytology from a dog with chronic bronchitis typically reveals a predominantly neutrophilic infiltrate with excessive mucus (**Fig. 3**). Small numbers of lymphocytes, eosinophils, goblet cells, ciliated cells, and epithelial cells and variable numbers of alveolar macrophages are also commonly observed. If a sample shows marked eosinophilia, eosinophilic bronchopneumopathy or parasitic infection (heartworm/ lung worm) should be considered. In Europe, the French heartworm (*Angiostrongylus*

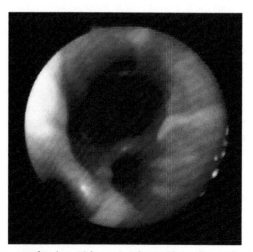

Fig. 2. Endoscopic image of a dog with severe chronic bronchitis. The epithelium is hyperemic and irregular. Copious mucus accumulation is apparent. (*Courtesy of* Dr Lynelle Johnson, DVM PhD, DACVIM (SA-IM), Davis, CA.)

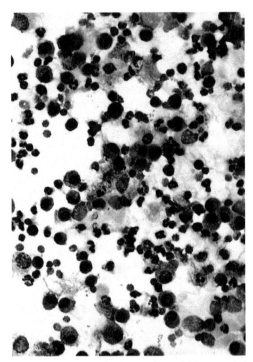

Fig. 3. Airway cytology from a dog with chronic bronchitis reveals increased neutrophils (53%, normal 5%–8%) as well as evidence of hemorrhage, mucin accumulation, and extracellular bacteria suggestive of contamination (Wright-Giemsa stain, original magnification 50×). (*Courtesy of* Dr Lynelle Johnson, DVM PhD, DACVIM (SA-IM), Davis, CA.)

vasorum) is a concern when airway eosinophilia is detected, and this infection has the potential to extend across North America in the future.[14]

Bacterial culture is commonly performed in association with airway cytology to rule out an infectious cause of cough. Detection of low numbers of bacteria is common but does not reflect true infection because the lower airways are not sterile. Positive bacterial cultures should be evaluated in light of the clinical appearance of a dog and in conjunction with observed cytology. For example, if cytology is largely acellular, with a few macrophages and an occasional neutrophil, yet microbiology isolates 1 + growth (or light growth) of a highly sensitive strain of *Escherichia coli*, it is unlikely that bacteria are playing a role in the clinical syndrome. In contrast, if cytology documents multiple degenerate neutrophils with intracellular bacteria, a positive bacterial culture provides useful information for treating that patient.

In people with chronic bronchitis, exacerbations associated with secondary bacterial infection are common, although they are not the primary cause of bronchitis. It is unclear whether this occurs in dogs with chronic bronchitis. *Mycoplasma* spp are incriminated as a respiratory pathogen, although this can be a fastidious organism to isolate using conventional bacteriologic techniques.[15] Polymerase chain reaction is useful in identifying the offending pathogen when appropriate primers are used. Pneumonia is a reasonable differential for cough; however, in contrast to dogs with chronic bronchitis, dogs with pneumonia are more commonly systemically unwell, with fever and lethargy; have a shorter duration of clinical signs; and more often display an alveolar infiltrate on thoracic radiographs.

PATHOPHYSIOLOGY

Chronic bronchitis results in inflammatory changes within the lower airways, including neutrophilic inflammation and evidence of increased mucus production. Bronchial wall thickening and malacia contribute to airflow obstruction and worsen development of inflammation. The inflammatory response also perpetuates coughing and contributes to progressive decline in lung function.

TREATMENT

If, after diagnostic testing, a clinical impression remains that a dog has chronic bronchitis, it is important to initiate therapy. Treatment goals for dogs with chronic bronchitis include reducing inflammation, limiting cough, and improving exercise stamina. Treatment also ideally prevents or slows disease progression and the associated airway remodeling.

Any environmental pollutants should be eliminated. Owners should be advised not to smoke indoors and to limit exposure of dogs to any airborne irritants. If extensive home remodeling with use of potentially noxious fumes is planned, consideration should be given to having a dog stay with friends or family. Exposure to potentially sick puppies should be avoided and trips to dog parks, grooming parlors, and boarding kennels should be limited to avoid development of infectious disease. Homes in humid climates can develop molds, and consultation with an air quality specialist could be considered if there is a high index of suspicion that molds or other pollutants are worsening clinical disease.

Obesity should be aggressively treated, because it markedly worsens cough and lung function and limits activity. A harness should be used in place of a collar, and episodes of excessive barking should be curtailed with appropriate behavior modification.

Glucocorticoids are the mainstay of treatment of CCB because they reduce inflammation, which reduces cough. Glucocorticoids are administered orally or via inhalation. Prednisone is the most commonly used glucocorticoid and is dosed at 1 to 2 mg/kg/d initially and then tapered to the lowest effective dose that controls clinical signs. For example, in a 10-kg dog with severe chronic bronchitis might be started on 10 mg of prednisone twice daily for 7 days or until cough is improved by 85% to 90%. Failure of the cough to improve should prompt consideration of an alternative diagnosis. After improvement, the dose could be decrease by 25% every 2 to 3 weeks until ideally the lowest possible dose is reached. Alternate-day therapy is preferred to allow normalization of the hypothalamic-pituitary axis and to limit clinical signs associated with use of exogenous glucocorticoids.

Inhaled glucocorticoids have been used widely in people and are used with growing frequency in dogs with CCB. Most dogs are easily trained to tolerate a face mask. One study demonstrated benefits of therapy with fluticasone (125 µg twice daily).[16] Inhaled steroids are delivered via a spacer chamber and face mask designed especially for dogs (eg, AeroDawg). Of clinical relevance, inhaled glucocorticoids are currently more expensive than oral glucocorticoids, although the systemic steroid-sparing effect can be worthwhile in improving quality of life. In the United States, fluticasone is available as 44 µg/puff, 110 µg/puff, and 220 µg/puff. The dosing approach is less clear in animals, because a substantial portion of the inhaled medication may not make it to the lungs/lower airways. A reasonable starting point is 10 to 20 µg/kg twice a day; rounded up to the available dose.

Bronchodilators are commonly prescribed for dogs with chronic bronchitis, although there is limited evidence of efficacy. Theophylline has been reported to have nonspecific effects that could be of benefit in CCB, such as decreasing diaphragmatic fatigue and increasing mucociliary clearance.[17] Extended-release theophylline administered at 10 mg/kg orally twice a day potentially improves expiratory airflow as well as enhances the efficacy of steroid treatment. β_2-Agonists, such as terbutaline, are thought less effective in dogs and can cause anxiety and restlessness.

Antibiotics are warranted in dogs with an acute exacerbation of chronic bronchitis and a reasonable suspicion of infection or in dogs with evidence of infection (neutrophils and bacteria) on tracheal wash cytology. Pending bacterial culture results, doxycycline (or less preferably minocycline) is a good choice for dogs with chronic bronchitis, as is azithromycin, because these drugs have anti-inflammatory properties as well as antimicrobial effects. Fluoroquinolones also have good respiratory penetration and could be useful in chronic bronchitis, although overuse of this class of drug leads to increased bacterial resistance. Concurrent administration of fluoroquinolones with theophylline can result in theophylline toxicity.[18]

Cough suppressants are helpful in CCB for improving the quality of life for dogs as well as for families. Additionally, ongoing cough promotes inflammation, which results in more cough. Therapy can be instituted when a clinician is reasonably comfortable that inflammation is acceptably controlled. Over-the-counter cough suppressants are rarely effective in dogs, and narcotic cough suppressants are most effective, with hydrocodone the most widely used (**Table 1**). A study in human medicine has just reported on the efficacy of gabapentin for control of cough in people, and this deserves investigation in dogs as well.[19]

PROGNOSIS

The clinical course of chronic bronchitis is variable. In the majority of dogs, there are permanent changes in the airways at the time of diagnosis, and the disease cannot be cured. Proper medical management typically ameliorates clinical signs and stops or slows progression of bronchial damage. Periodic relapses of cough are not uncommon and require adjustments in the treatment protocol, such as a temporary increase in glucocorticoids or addition of bronchodilators, antibiotics, or cough suppressants, until improvement in clinical signs.

PULMONARY HYPERTENSION

Pulmonary hypertension, defined as a systolic pulmonary arterial pressure greater than 25 mm Hg at rest can develop in dogs with chronic bronchitis. Chronic pulmonary disease results in pulmonary hypertension in part due to hypoxic pulmonary vasoconstriction leading to permanent medial hypertrophy. Release of inflammatory mediators or

Table 1		
Cough suppressants used in canine chronic bronchitis. Opioids may be titrated up as needed, although tolerance can result. Side effects are primarily excessive sedation		
Drug	**Dose**	**Comments**
Opioids (most effective)		
Butorphanol	0.25–1.1 mg/kg q 8–12 h	Expensive; titrate upwards
Hydrocodone	0.2–0.3 mg/kg q 6–12 h	—
Tramadol	2–5 mg/kg po q 8–12 h	Less effective, inexpensive
Nonopioids (less effective)		
Gabapentin	2–5 mg/kg po q 8	Unestablished efficacy
Methocarbamol	15–30 mg/kg q 12	Unestablished efficacy

vasoconstrictive agents (eg, endothelin), however, might also play a role. Pulmonary hypertension is associated with exercise intolerance and progressive pulmonary dysfunction. The percentage of dogs with chronic bronchitis that develop pulmonary hypertension is unknown, but it should be considered in dogs with CCB that display syncope or severe exercise intolerance. Pulmonary hypertension is most often documented by Doppler interrogation of the tricuspid (or pulmonary valve) with determination of the velocity of regurgitant flow, which permits an estimate of pulmonary arterial pressure.[20] Although treatment of chronic bronchitis should continue, pulmonary hypertension in dogs is treated most effectively at this time with sildenafil or other competitive inhibitors of phosphodiesterase type 5.[21] The recommended oral dosage for sildenafil is 2 to 5 mg/kg every 8 hours. Titrate to the lowest effective dose. Side effects of higher doses are hypotension. Sildenafil should not be combined with nitrates.

WHAT TO DO WHEN THE DOG IS STILL COUGHING?

Persistent or poorly responsive cough is frustrating for clients, veterinarians, and likely dogs. In dogs with a confirmed diagnosis of chronic bronchitis that are presenting with recurrent or worsening cough, it is worthwhile to confirm that dog and owner have been compliant with the prescribed medications because small dogs in particular are often difficult to medicate. Additionally, it is prudent to re-evaluate the diagnosis via auscultation and thoracic radiographs. Congestive heart failure could develop in dogs with progressive mitral valve disease, and other diseases, such as pneumonia, pulmonary neoplasia, or pulmonary fibrosis, can develop. In dogs without apparent confounding disease, one option to control cough is increasing the dose and frequency of administration of a cough suppressant until the dog is heavily sedated for at least 12 to 24 hours to limit inflammation that perpetuates cough. In rare cases, the author has used fentanyl patches for short-term control of cough. Additionally, in people, and likely in dogs with exacerbations, antibiotics are often helpful in reducing bacterial colonization of diseased airways. Finally, increasing prednisone or administering parenteral glucocorticoids is often useful. When clinical signs abate, the dose is tapered back to a lower dose. In some cases, hospitalizing a dog for supplemental oxygen permits the dog's signs to improve and additionally allow owners a night of uninterrupted sleep, which can increase their enthusiasm and tolerance for treating the dog.

SUMMARY

CCB is a common cause of chronic cough and is a condition that frequently is treated by practicing clinicians. A sound understanding of the pathophysiology, diagnosis, and treatment of the condition allows for prolonged quality of life for patients. Owner education of dogs with chronic bronchitis is essential because CCB is a progressive, chronic disease. Treatment can ameliorate clinical signs, but ongoing airway disease and some form of cough likely persist. Frequent checkups and tailoring of a therapeutic plan to individual dogs provide the best outcome. Advancement in methods for early detection of chronic bronchitis and more effective treatments will improve understanding of this disease and allow limiting the long-term effects it has on dogs.

REFERENCES

1. Johnson LR, Queen EV, Vernau W, et al. Microbiologic and cytologic assessment of bronchoalveolar lavage fluid from dogs with lower respiratory tract infection: 105 cases (2001-2011). J Vet Intern Med 2013;27:259–67.

2. Stanley BJ, Hauptman JG, Fritz MC, et al. Esophageal dysfunction in dogs with idiopathic laryngeal paralysis: a controlled cohort study. Vet Surg 2010;39(2): 139–49.

3. Lux CN, Archer TM, Lunsford KV. Gastroesophageal reflux and laryngeal dysfunction in a dog. J Am Vet Med Assoc 2012;240:1100–3.

4. Madanick RD. Management of GERD-Related Chronic Cough. Gastroenterol Hepatol (N Y) 2013;9:311–3.

5. Poncet CM, Dupre GP, Freiche VG, et al. Prevalence of gastrointestinal tract lesions in 73 brachycephalic dogs with upper respiratory syndrome. J Small Anim Pract 2005;46:273–9.

6. Singh MK, Johnson LR, Kittleson MD, et al. Bronchomalacia in dogs with myxomatous mitral valve degeneration. J Vet Intern Med 2012;26:312–9.

7. Hawkins EC, Basseches J, Berry CR, et al. Demographic, clinical, and radiographic features of bronchiectasis in dogs: 316 cases (1988-2000). J Am Vet Med Assoc 2003;223:1628–35.

8. Hawkins EC, Clay LD, Bradley JM, et al. Demographic and historical findings, including exposure to environmental tobacco smoke, in dogs with chronic cough. J Vet Intern Med 2010;24:825–31.

9. Oyama MA, Rush JE, Rozanski EA. Assessment of serum N-terminal pro-B-type natriuretic peptide concentration for differentiation of congestive heart failure from primary respiratory tract disease as the cause of respiratory signs in dogs. J Am Vet Med Assoc 2009;235(11):1319–25.

10. Padrid PA, Hornof WJ, Kurpershoek CJ, et al. Canine chronic bronchitis: a pathophysiologic evaluation of 18 cases. J Vet Intern Med 1990;4:172–80.

11. Swimmer RA, Rozanski EA. Evaluation of the 6-minute walk test in pet dogs. J Vet Intern Med 2011;25:405–6.

12. Brownlie SE. A retrospective study of diagnosis in 109 cases of canine lower respiratory disease. J Small Anim Pract 1990;31:371–6.

13. Creevy KE. Airway evaluation and flexible endoscopic procedures in dogs and cats: laryngoscopy, transtracheal wash, tracheobronchoscopy, and bronchoalveolar lavage. Vet Clin North Am Small Anim Pract 2009;39:869–80.

14. Conboy GA. Canine angiostrongylosis: the French heartworm: an emerging threat in North America. Vet Parasitol 2011;176:382–9.

15. Chandler JC, Lappin MR. Mycoplasmal respiratory infections in small animals: 17 Cases (1988-1999). J Am Anim Hosp Assoc 2002;38:111–9.

16. Bexfield NH, Foale RD, Davison LJ, et al. Management of 13 cases of canine respiratory disease using inhaled corticosteroids. J Small Anim Pract 2006;47: 377–82.

17. Bach JF, Kukanich B, Papich MG, et al. Evaluation of the bioavailability and pharmacokinetics of two extended-release theophylline formulation in dogs. J Am Vet Med Assoc 2004;224:1113–9.

18. Antoniou T, Gomes T, Mamdani MM, et al. Ciprofloxacin-induced theophylline toxicity: a population-based study. Eur J Clin Pharmacol 2011;67(5):521–6.

19. Ryan NM, Birring SS, Gibson PG. Gabapentin for refractory chronic cough: a randomised, double-blind, placebo-controlled trial. Lancet 2012;380(9853): 1583–9.

20. Johnson L, Boon J, Orton EC. Clinical characteristics of 53 dogs with Doppler-derived evidence of pulmonary hypertension: 1992-1996. J Vet Intern Med 1999;13:440–7.

21. Brown AJ, Davison E, Sleeper MM. Clinical efficacy of sildenafil in treatment of pulmonary arterial hypertension in dogs. J Vet Intern Med 2010;24:850–4.

Tracheal and Airway Collapse in Dogs

Ann Della Maggiore, DVM

KEYWORDS

- Tracheal collapse • Airway collapse • Bronchomalacia • Chronic cough
- Tracheal stent

KEY POINTS

- Tracheal collapse is characterized by dorsoventral flattening of tracheal rings.
- Tracheal collapse affects the cervical and/or intrathoracic trachea and is seen most commonly in middle-aged to older toy and miniature breed dogs.
- Airway collapse or bronchomalacia affects large bronchi that contain cartilage and could be associated with similar cartilage defects to those seen with tracheal collapse.
- Medical management can include reduction of stress, weight loss, antitussives, bronchodilators, and possibly glucocorticoids and antibiotics.
- Surgical and minimally invasive treatment options are available when medical management fails.

INTRODUCTION

Tracheal or airway collapse is a common cause of cough in dogs and can affect the cervical trachea, intrathoracic trachea, or bronchial walls in isolation, or multiple regions can be affected concurrently. Tracheal collapse results from softening of the tracheal cartilage. It is typically characterized by dorsoventral flattening of the tracheal rings and prolapse of the tracheal membrane into the lumen. This prolapse leads to narrowing of the trachea whenever extraluminal pressure exceeds intraluminal pressure, causing airway collapse and impeding the passage of air. Clinically this results in a persistent dry, paroxysmal "goose-honk" cough, tracheal sensitivity, and varying degrees of respiratory difficulty. When the principal bronchi are also involved, the condition is termed tracheobronchomalacia. Bronchomalacia, which is recognized in people and in dogs, is a defect of the principal bronchi and other smaller airways supported by cartilage that causes narrowing and loss of luminal dimensions in intrathoracic airways and a reduction in ability to clear secretions. These changes result in bronchial collapse, causing chronic cough, wheezing, and intermittent or chronic respiratory difficulty.[1,2]

Disclosures: None.
William R. Pritchard Veterinary Medical Teaching Hospital, University of California–Davis, Small Animal Internal Medicine, 1 Shields Avenue, Davis, CA 95616, USA
E-mail address: adellamaggiore@ucdavis.edu

Vet Clin Small Anim 44 (2014) 117–127
http://dx.doi.org/10.1016/j.cvsm.2013.09.004
0195-5616/14/$ – see front matter © 2014 Elsevier Inc. All rights reserved.

CAUSE/PATHOPHYSIOLOGY

The cause of malacic airway disease is complex, incompletely understood, and likely multifactorial. In people, proposed causes include congenital conditions, endotracheal intubation, long-term ventilation, closed-chest trauma, chronic airway irritation and inflammation, malignancy, asthma, mechanical anatomic factors, and thyroid disease, but a definitive cause is unknown.[3–12] The cause of tracheobronchomalacia in dogs is also unknown and could be primary (congenital) or secondary to chronic inflammation (acquired). Given the common occurrence of tracheal collapse in small breed dogs, there could be a primary or congenital abnormality of cartilage with secondary factors playing a role in progression and development of clinical signs.

Tracheal collapse is associated with softening of cartilage rings due to a reduction of glycosaminoglycan and chondroitin sulfate, which leads to a weakness and flattening of the tracheal rings. Changes to the tracheal matrix and an inability to retain water lead to a decreased ability to maintain functional rigidity.[13,14] Extrinsic compression, chronic inflammation, and alteration in elastic fibers in the dorsal tracheal membrane and annular ligaments have also been considered as possible causes or factors that contribute to collapse.[15,16] Secondary factors that can initiate clinical signs include airway irritants, chronic bronchitis, laryngeal paralysis, respiratory infection, obesity, and tracheal intubation. It is critical to identify these factors for appropriate medical management.

Dynamic collapse of the airway perpetuates additional inflammation, tracheal edema, alterations or failure in the mucociliary apparatus, increased mucus secretion, and mucus trapping within the airways. The cervical trachea will collapse during inspiration and the thoracic trachea will collapse during expiration due to the pressures developed during the respiratory cycle. Tracheal collapse occurs almost exclusively in small breed dogs, while bronchial collapse occurs in both large and small breed dogs and most commonly involves the right middle and the left cranial bronchi.[1] In some dogs only bronchial collapse (bronchomalacia) is noted.

PATIENT HISTORY

Tracheal collapse is commonly seen in middle-aged to older miniature, toy, and small breed dogs. Age at presentation typically ranges from 1 to 15 years and signs have been present for years, although about 25% of affected dogs show clinical signs by the age of 6 months.[17] Breeds overrepresented include Yorkshire terriers, Pomeranian, Pugs, Poodle, Maltese, and Chihuahuas.[18] No sex predilection has been appreciated. Cats and large breed dogs are rarely diagnosed with tracheal collapse.

Bronchomalacia is reported in 45% to 83% of dogs with tracheal collapse[1,19] and has also been reported in dogs with eosinophilic bronchopneumopathy[20] or bronchitis. Bronchomalacia, unlike tracheal collapse, can affect any canine breed and can be seen in medium- and large- breed dogs,[1,2] suggesting that the underlying cause could be different from tracheal collapse, although histologic investigations are lacking. Within a population of coughing dogs, dogs with airway collapse are often older and lower in body weight, and have a significantly higher body condition than dogs without airway collapse.[1] Bronchomalacia and, specifically, collapse of the left cranial lobar bronchus, has been recognized in a large percentage (87%) of dogs with brachycephalic airway syndrome. In one report, Pugs were the most common brachycephalic breed affected with bronchomalacia, followed by English Bulldogs and French Bulldogs.[21]

Dogs with tracheal or airway collapse usually present to the veterinarian for evaluation of cough that is initiated by excitement, drinking or eating, or pulling on a leash with a neck lead. Prolonged clinical history is common and ranges from weeks to years, although some dogs present at a very young age with respiratory distress due to airway narrowing and obstruction. Dogs typically have paroxysmal or waxing and waning respiratory signs, most often described as a dry, harsh, or "honking" cough. Worsening tachypnea, exercise intolerance, and respiratory distress tend to occur during physical exertion or heat stress or in humid conditions. Respiratory compromise can progress and become refractory to treatment. Cyanosis and syncope can also occur because of complete airway obstruction, vagally mediated syncope, or pulmonary hypertension.[22]

PHYSICAL EXAMINATION

Dogs presenting for airway collapse are usually systemically healthy and are often overweight. Respiratory pattern is often normal or the dog can show increased respiratory effort due to airway collapse. Cervical tracheal collapse typically causes respiratory difficulty on inspiration, whereas intrathoracic collapse and bronchomalacia result in increased expiratory effort. Close observation at the thoracic inlet can sometimes reveal cranial lung herniation through the inlet during expiration in some dogs with intrathoracic airway collapse. Palpation of the trachea frequently initiates cough in affected dogs, indicating nonspecific tracheal sensitivity. Palpation should be performed cautiously as some animals will become cyanotic, develop syncope, or go into a life-threatening respiratory crisis due to paroxysmal cough. Collapse of the cervical trachea can sometimes be appreciated as a flattening of the tracheal rings on cervical palpation.

Auscultation over the trachea can reveal stridorous sounds on both inspiration and expiration due to the fixed narrowing of the extrathoracic tracheal diameter and must be differentiated from laryngeal paralysis, which is reported in up to 60% of dogs with tracheal collapse,[22] emphasizing the importance of a thorough upper airway examination if the animal is anesthetized. Stertor or stridor could also indicate laryngeal collapse in brachycephalic breeds, with one study reporting some degree of laryngeal collapse in almost all brachycephalic dogs as well as an association between laryngeal collapse and collapse of the left cranial lobar bronchus.[21] During thoracic auscultation, referred upper airway sounds are often noted and can compromise assessment of lung sounds. Crackles on both inspiration and expiration are sometimes appreciated in dogs with bronchomalacia and small airway collapse, or this can suggest mucus accumulation in the airways associated with concurrent bronchitis.

A thorough cardiac auscultation is recommended, and a heart murmur associated with mitral regurgitation was found significantly more often in dogs with airway collapse (17%) when compared with animals presenting with cough without airway collapse (2%).[1] Airway collapse most likely is related to the commonality of myxomatous mitral regurgitation and airway disease in small breed dogs. The role of cardiomegaly and specifically left atrial enlargement in airway collapse remains unclear. A recent study showed similar severity and location of airway collapse in dogs with and without left atrial enlargement and reported airway inflammation as the likely cause of cough in dogs that had both left atrial enlargement and airway collapse.[23]

Hepatomegaly is common in dogs with tracheal collapse and could be a reflection of obesity, although hepatic dysfunction (as indicated by elevations in bile acids) has been reported in dogs with tracheal collapse.[24]

DIAGNOSTIC EVALUATION
Hematologic, Biochemical Evaluation, and Heartworm Screening

The diagnosis of tracheal collapse is strongly suspected based on signalment, history of cough, and physical examination findings. Additional diagnostic evaluation should be performed to rule out concurrent disorders and determine appropriate therapy.

A complete blood count, chemistry panel, and heartworm screening are recommended in any coughing dog before additional diagnostic evaluation. These results are typically unremarkable in dogs with airway collapse, although evaluation of dogs with severe tracheal collapse showed that 12 of 26 dogs had elevations in 2 or more liver enzymes, and stimulated bile acids were elevated in 25 of 26 dogs. Following stent placement for management of severe, refractory airway obstruction, bile acid concentrations decreased but plasma liver enzyme activity was not significantly influenced.[24] The cause of these changes remains unknown, although hypoxia and development of a centrilobular liver cell necrosis were suggested as possible causes of liver dysfunction, similar to what has been reported in humans with acute exacerbation of chronic respiratory disease.

Thoracic and Cervical Radiographs

Detection and grading of tracheal collapse is used to identify the location and severity of collapse and to monitor progression of the disease. Because tracheal and airway collapse are considered dynamic processes, it is ideal to perform diagnostic imaging in multiple stages of the respiratory cycle. Collapse of the cervical trachea should be evident on inspiration and the intrathoracic trachea will collapse on expiration. It is recommended to evaluate a lateral radiograph of the thorax and cervical region (**Fig. 1**) in both the inspiratory and the expiratory phases, although this only slightly improves accuracy in the detection of collapse.[18] False positives and false negatives are common with plain radiography. Radiographs often underestimate the frequency and severity of tracheal collapse and often fail to detect collapse at the carina, which is reportedly more severe than cervical collapse.[18]

Fluoroscopy

A fluoroscopic study can be used to evaluate a coughing dog for the presence and location of airway collapse but this technique is only available at universities and large referral hospitals. When radiography was compared with fluoroscopy, assuming the fluoroscopy was correct, radiographic evidence of collapse was at the incorrect location in 44% of dogs and it was not detected in 8% of dogs with radiographs alone.[18] Fluoroscopic identification of lower airway collapse versus tracheal collapse can be important in determining therapy (see treatment) (**Fig. 2**).

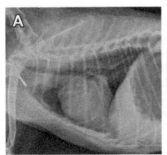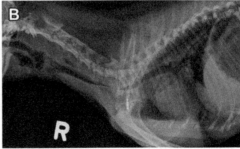

Fig. 1. Lateral thoracic (*A*) and cervical (*B*) radiographs of a dog with cervical tracheal collapse at the thoracic inlet. Note that the additional view (*B*) improves the ability to identify cervical tracheal collapse. Retraction of the larynx in (*B*) likely reflects upper airway obstruction. (*Courtesy of* Lynelle Johnson, DVM, MS, PhD, DACVIM, Davis, CA.)

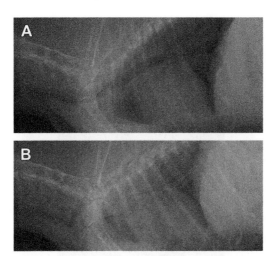

Fig. 2. Images captured from a fluoroscopic study on inspiration (*A*) and expiration (*B*) from a dog with intrathoracic tracheal collapse clearly show the change in luminal diameter of the intrathoracic airway during expiration. (*Courtesy of* Lynelle Johnson, DVM, MS, PhD, DACVIM, Davis, CA.)

Bronchoscopy

Bronchoscopy is considered the gold standard for diagnosis of bronchomalacia in humans because it allows visualization of the trachea and the principal, lobar, and sublobar bronchi to assess for bronchomalacia.[25] In addition to bronchoscopy, laryngoscopy and bronchoalveolar lavage are recommended in coughing dogs to detect concurrent disease that affect treatment. Bronchoscopy does require anesthesia, which can be associated with complications in animals with severe airway obstruction, marked tracheal sensitivity, dramatic expiratory effort, or in those that are obese or overly excitable.

Laryngeal collapse and paralysis can be seen concurrently with tracheal collapse and bronchomalacia; therefore, a thorough upper airway evaluation is recommended and should be performed before intubation at anesthetic induction. Laryngeal collapse is graded in 3 stages based on severity.[26] Stage 1 is characterized by eversion of the laryngeal saccules; stage 2 is characterized by medial displacement of the cuneiform process of the arytenoid cartilages, and stage 3 is characterized by collapse of the corniculate processes of the arytenoid cartilages with the loss of the dorsal arch of the rima glottis. See the article on Laryngeal disease by MacPail elsewhere in this issue for further details. As mentioned previously, in one report, laryngeal collapse was significantly correlated with severe bronchial collapse in brachycephalic dogs.[21]

Bronchoscopic examination should be performed in a standardized fashion with the use of tracheal bronchial anatomy and nomenclature as proposed by Amis and McKiernan[27] for proper identification. Grading of tracheal collapse is based on a scheme determined by Tagner and Hobson[28] related to the reduction in luminal dimension (**Fig. 3, Table 1**).

Bronchoscopy also allows evaluation of the principal and lobar bronchi for evidence of bronchomalacia and identifies specific segments of bronchial collapse. Bronchial collapse in both brachycephalic and nonbrachycephalic dogs most commonly involves the left cranial and right middle bronchi.[2,3,21,23] In one study, 48% of dogs diagnosed with bronchomalacia had concurrent tracheal collapse,[3] whereas in another,[1]

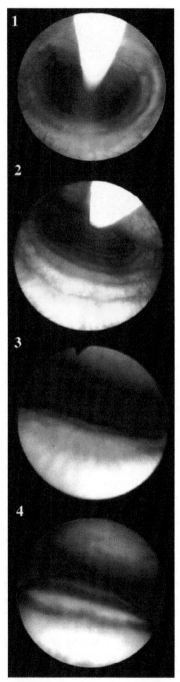

Fig. 3. Grades of tracheal collapse. (*From* Johnson LR, Pollard RE. Tracheal collapse and bronchomalacia in dogs: 58 cases (7/2001-1/2008). J Vet Intern Med 2010;24:298–305; with permission.)

Table 1	
Grading of tracheal collapse	
Grade	Reduction in Luminal Diameter (%)
1	25
2	50
3	75
4	90–100 (obstruction of lumen or a double-lumen trachea)

41% had tracheal collapse in conjunction with bronchial collapse. In dogs with collapse of sublobar airways, focal airway collapse was identified in 48% and diffuse airway collapse was present in 52% of dogs.[1] Bronchomalacia commonly goes under-diagnosed because it is not visible radiographically and endoscopy is required for definitive diagnosis.

In humans bronchomalacia and dynamic airway collapse are defined as 2 separate entities, and until recently, had not been investigated in dogs. Normal airways are recognized as round or ovoid with minimal luminal variation (subjectively <20%) during the respiratory cycle.[1] A recent study examined clinical evaluation and endoscopic classification of bronchomalacia in dogs and provided evidence that static and dynamic bronchomalacia seem to occur both independently and concurrently. Dynamic bronchial collapse was found alone in 59% of cases or with static bronchial collapse in 37% of dogs, and most animals (71%) had dynamic bronchial collapse and tracheal collapse.[3] Bronchial collapse in that study was defined as static if a stable airway diameter was seen or dynamic if changes in luminal diameter were noted during respiration (**Fig. 4**). A grading system was developed with grade I collapse defined as static or dynamic collapse with reduction in diameter less than or equal to 50%, grade 2 collapse as diameter reduction greater than 50% and less than or equal to 75%, and grade 3 collapse as greater than 75%, with contact between the dorsal and ventral mucosa of the collapsed bronchus.[3] If use of this grading system becomes widespread, prospective studies could be designed to assess progression of disease and better establish prognosis, as well as guidelines for therapeutic intervention.

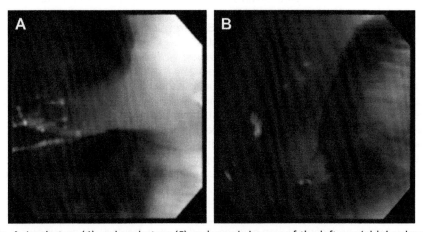

Fig. 4. Inspiratory (A) and expiratory (B) endoscopic images of the left cranial lobar bronchus in a dog with bronchomalacia. (*Courtesy of* Lynelle Johnson, DVM, MS, PhD, DACVIM, Davis, CA.)

Common bronchoscopic findings in some dogs with airway collapse include gross evidence of airway inflammation, hyperemia, and mucus accumulation. Bronchoalveolar lavage cytology is used to document infectious or inflammatory conditions, and culture is used to rule out concurrent infection. Varying types of inflammation have been identified in dogs with airway collapse, although a previous study comparing dogs with airway collapse and dogs without airway collapse showed no clear differences in airway inflammation between groups.[1] In animals with bronchomalacia that have had bronchoalveolar lavage performed, neutrophilic inflammation was found in 51%.[3] In dogs with airway collapse and left atrial enlargement, both neutrophilic and lymphocytic were commonly identified.[21] It remains unclear whether inflammation precedes or follows airway collapse.

TREATMENT

The approach to treatment of airway collapse varies with the location of collapse and the severity of the animal's clinical signs. An animal presenting in respiratory distress is a medical emergency and requires stabilization before diagnostic testing. Stress should be minimized and oxygen provided as flow-by or in an oxygen cage. Acepromazine (0.01–0.1 mg/kg SC every 4–6 hours) and butorphanol (0.05–0.1 mg/kg SC every 4–6 hours) can be synergistic in providing sedation and cough suppression, but caution should be used as oversedation could make intubation necessary. Dogs should be maintained in a cool environment because patients with upper airway obstructions are predisposed to hyperthermia. Glucocorticoids are sometimes necessary to decrease laryngeal inflammation or edema. Once the dog is stabilized, additional diagnostics and treatment options can be considered.

MEDICAL MANAGEMENT
Environmental Factors

As an adjunct to medical therapy, environmental changes should be instituted to maintain the animal in a cool environment with minimal humidity. An owner's ability to recognize and reduce specific environmental factors that increase barking, anxiety, and excitement can help decrease the stimulus to cough. Using a harness instead of a neck collar reduces direct stimulation and compression of the trachea.

Encouraging weight loss is one of the single most essential strategies for reducing clinical signs in dogs with airway collapse. By increasing thoracic wall compliance and reducing extrathoracic and intra-abdominal adipose tissue, cough and respiratory difficulty can be substantially reduced. However, weight loss is typically challenging because many of these dogs cannot effectively exercise. Careful diet planning is essential. Current caloric intake from all sources should be determined and resting energy requirement calculated through the formula: $RER = 70 \times (BW)^{0.75}$ (RER: resting energy requirement; BW:body weight in kg). It is important that owners are given realistic expectations for weight loss, and ideally, a dog will lose 1% to 2% weight per week. Caloric restriction alone is used initially with weekly monitoring of weight. If this is unsuccessful, a prescription diet comprising a low-calorie, high-fiber diet should be used. Identification and treatment of secondary medical conditions are also important for appropriate management.

Antitussive Agents

When infection and inflammation have been adequately treated, cough suppressants are recommended to reduce chronic irritation and control cough. Cough suppressants are often the sole therapy used for cough associated with cervical tracheal collapse.

Cough suppressants regularly used include hydrocodone (0.22 mg/kg PO 2 to 4 times a day) and butorphanol (0.55 mg/kg PO 2 to 4 times a day). When treating an animal with cough suppressants, it is recommended to start at a frequent dosing interval and gradually prolong the time between dose administration until the lowest effective dose is used at the longest interval. Side effects of these drugs include sedation, constipation, and development of tolerance.

Glucocorticoids

Glucocorticoids are often used short term to reduce laryngeal, tracheal, and bronchial inflammation, unless a concurrent infectious condition is suspected. Initial treatment typically involves an anti-inflammatory dose of prednisone (0.5 mg/kg PO 2 times a day) or inhaled steroids (fluticasone propionate, 110 μg/puff, administered via face mask and spacing chamber) for 5 to 7 days. A short course of therapy is advised to avoid secondary effects such as panting, which puts added stress on the respiratory system, and weight gain. Use of inhaled corticosteroids in place of systemic can be used to minimize side effects.

Bronchodilators

Bronchodilators are sometimes used when small airway disease is suspected to contribute to intrathoracic airway collapse. Use is based on the theory that any increase in diameter of small (<300 μm) airways will improve expiratory airflow, alter pressure dynamics, and reduce the tendency for intrathoracic airway to collapse. Bronchodilators have no effect on larger airways that are visible during endoscopy and are not indicated for treatment of cervical tracheal collapse. Bronchodilators can play an important role when lower airway collapse/bronchomalacia is suspected or documented on bronchoscopic evaluation, although response is variable. Methylxanthine bronchodilators are most commonly used and extended-release theophylline is recommended at 10 mg/kg PO every 12 hours. Tablets can usually be cut in half and extended-release capabilities maintained. β_2-Agonists are more effective as true bronchodilators but do not seem to be as useful in management of airway collapse.

Antibiotics

Infection rarely contributes to clinical signs in airway collapse, but antibiotics can play an important role in treating secondary infections that act as an inciting cause to airway irritation. Doxycycline can be considered pending culture results for treatment of *Mycoplasma* infection as well as for anti-inflammatory effects.

Surgical Management

When medical management fails to control clinical signs, surgical intervention or placement of an intraluminal stent should be considered. Extraluminal tracheal rings are indicated for cervical tracheal collapse and excellent outcomes have been reported in dogs managed by skilled surgeons.[29] Postoperative laryngeal paralysis can be anticipated as a potential problem because of impingement or praxis of the recurrent laryngeal nerve, and if stridor or inspiratory respiratory distress occurs after placement of extraluminal rings, laryngeal lateralization is generally needed. Tracheal necrosis can also be encountered long term if blood supply is damaged.[30–32]

If intrathoracic tracheal collapse is diagnosed and cannot be managed medically, placement of an intraluminal stent can be considered. Intraluminal stents can be life-saving and excellent short- and long-term outcomes have been reported.[19,33]

Extensive medical management is often required to control cough, infection, and inflammation postoperatively. Complications include bacterial tracheitis, stent fracture/migration, and development of obstructive granulation tissue.

Prognosis

Little has been published about overall prognosis in dogs with airway collapse that are medically managed. There is concern that disease will gradually progress over time and dogs will become refractory to treatment. However, most dogs can be successfully managed with diligent attention to weight control, identification and control of infection and inflammation, and appropriate use of interventional therapy.

REFERENCES

1. Johnson LR, Pollard RE. Tracheal collapse and bronchomalacia in dogs: 58 cases (7/2001-1/2008). J Vet Intern Med 2010;24:298–305.
2. Adamama-Moraitou KK, Pardali D, Day MJ, et al. Canine bronchomalacia: a clinicopathological study of 18 cases diagnosed by endoscopy. Vet J 2012;191(2): 261–6.
3. Bottero E, Bellino C, De Lorenzi D, et al. Clinical evaluation and endoscopic classification of bronchomalacia in dogs. J Vet Intern Med 2013;27(4):840–6.
4. Mair E, Parsons DS. Pediatric tracheomalacia and major airway collapse. Ann Otol Rhinol Laryngol 1992;101:300–9.
5. Feist JH, Johnson TH, Wilson RJ. Acquired tracheomalacia: etiology and differential diagnosis. Chest 1975;68:340–5.
6. Burden RJ, Shann F, Butt W, et al. Tracheobronchial malacia and stenosis in children in intensive care: bronchograms help to predict outcome. Thorax 1999;54: 511–7.
7. Tsugawa C, Nishijima E, Muraji T, et al. A shape memory airway stent for tracheomalacia in children: an experimental and clinical study. J Pediatr Surg 1997;32: 50–3.
8. Johnson TH, Mikita J, Wilson RJ, et al. Acquired tracheomalacia. Radiology 1973; 109:576–80.
9. Tillie-Lebold I, Wallaert B, Leblond D, et al. Respiratory involvement in relapsing polychondritis. Clinical, functional, endoscopic, and radiographic evaluations. Medicine 1998;77:168–76.
10. Miyazawa T, Miyazu Y, Iwamoto Y, et al. Stenting at the flow-limiting segment in tracheobronchial stenosis due to lung cancer. Am J Respir Crit Care Med 2004;169:1096–102.
11. Nuutinen J. Acquired tracheobronchomalacia. Eur J Respir Dis 1982;63: 380–7.
12. McHenry CR, Pitrowski JJ. Thyroidectomy in patients with marked thyroid enlargement: airway management, morbidity, and outcome. Am Surg 1994;60: 586–91.
13. Dallman MJ, McClure RC, Brown EM. Normal and collapsed trachea in the dog. Scanning electron microscopy study. Am J Vet Res 1985;46(10):2110–5.
14. Dallman MJ, McClure RC, Brown EM. Histochemical study of normal and collapsed tracheas in dogs. Am J Vet Res 1988;49(12):2117–25.
15. Jokinen K, Palva T, Sutinen S, et al. Acquired tracheobronchomalacia. Ann Clin Res 1977;9:52–7.
16. Kamanta S, Usui N, Sawai T, et al. Pexis of the great vessels for patients with tracheobronchomalacia in infancy. J Pediatr Surg 2000;35:454–7.

17. Herrtage MJ. Medical management of tracheal collapse. In: Bonagura J, Twedt D, editors. Kirks current veterinary therapy XIV. St Louis (MO): Saunders Elsevier; 2009. p. 630–5.
18. Macready DM, Johnson LR, Pollard RE. Fluoroscopic and radiographic evaluation of tracheal collapse in 62 dogs. J Am Vet Med Assoc 2007;230:1870–6.
19. Moritz A, Schneider M, Bauer N. Management of advanced tracheal collapse in dogs using intraluminal self-expanding biliary wall stents. J Vet Intern Med 2004; 18:31–42.
20. Clercx C, Peeters D, Snaps F, et al. Eosinophilic bronchopneumopathy in dogs. J Vet Intern Med 2000;14:282–91.
21. De Lorenzi D, Bertoncello D, Drigo M. Bronchial abnormalities found in a consecutive series of forty brachycephalic dogs. J Am Vet Med Assoc 2009;235:835–40.
22. Johnson LR. Diseases of airways. In: Johnson L, editor. Clinical canine and feline respiratory medicine. Ames (IA): Wiley-Blackwell Publishing; 2010. p. 97–103.
23. Singh MK, Johnson LR, Kittleson MD, et al. Bronchomalacia in dogs with myxomatous mitral valve degeneration. J Vet Intern Med 2012;26:312–9.
24. Bauer NB, Schneider MA, Neiger R, et al. Liver disease in dogs with tracheal collapse. J Vet Intern Med 2006;20:845–9.
25. Heyer CM, Nuesslein TG, Jung D, et al. Tracheobronchial anomalies and stenoses: detection with low-dose multidetector CT with virtual tracheobronchoscopy-comparison with flexible tracheobronchoscopy. Radiology 2007;242:542–9.
26. Leonard HC. Collapse of the larynx and associated structures in the dog. J Am Vet Med Assoc 1960;137:360–3.
27. Amis TC, McKiernan BM. Systemic identification of endobronchial anatomy during bronchoscopy in the dog. Am J Vet Res 1986;47:2649–57.
28. Tangner CH, Hobson HP. A retrospective study of 20 surgically managed cases of collapsed trachea. Vet Surg 1982;11:146–9.
29. Buback JL, Boothe HW, Hobson HP. Surgical treatment of tracheal collapse in dogs; 90 cases (1983-1993). J Am Vet Med Assoc 1996;208(3):380–4.
30. White RN. Unilateral arytenoid lateralization and extraluminal polypropylene ring prosthesis for correction of tracheal collapse in the dog. J Small Anim Pract 1995; 36:151–8.
31. Kirby BM, Bjorling DE, Rankin JH, et al. The effects of surgical isolation and application of polypropylene spiral prosthese on tracheal blood flow. Vet Surg 1992; 20:49–54.
32. Coyne BE, Fingland RB, Kennedy GA, et al. Clinical and pathologic effects of a modified technique for application of spiral prosthese to the cervical trachea of dogs. Vet Surg 1993;22:269–75.
33. Sura PA, Krahwinkel DJ. Self-expanding nitinol stents for the treatment of tracheal collapse in dogs: 12 cases (2001-2004). J Am Vet Med Assoc 2008;232:228–36.

Idiopathic Pulmonary Fibrosis in West Highland White Terriers

Henna P. Heikkilä-Laurila, DVM*, Minna M. Rajamäki, DVM, PhD

KEYWORDS

- Dog • Interstitial lung disease • Bronchoalveolar lavage • Arterial blood gases
- HRCT • Biomarker

KEY POINTS

- Canine idiopathic pulmonary fibrosis (CIPF) is a chronic, progressive, interstitial lung disease of unknown cause affecting mainly middle-aged and old West Highland white terriers.
- Typical findings are cough, exercise intolerance, Velcro crackles, an abdominal breathing pattern, and hypoxemia.
- Bronchial changes are present in many dogs and bronchoalveolar lavage fluid analysis usually shows an increased total cell count.
- Diagnosis is one of exclusion and often requires either high-resolution CT imaging or histopathology of the lung tissue, which is seldom performed on living dogs.
- CIPF shares several clinical findings with human idiopathic pulmonary fibrosis (IPF); however, in histopathology, CIPF has features of human IPF but also of human nonspecific interstitial pneumonia.
- No effective treatment exists, but corticosteroids and theophylline can ease clinical signs in dogs. Pirfenidone is the only licensed drug to treat IPF in humans, but it does not result in cure.

INTRODUCTION

Idiopathic pulmonary fibrosis (IPF) is a chronic, progressive interstitial lung disease (ILD) of unknown cause.[1] The disease is recognized in humans,[1,2] cats,[3,4] and dogs.[5–8] The prevalence and incidence of canine IPF (CIPF) are currently unknown and can be difficult to estimate. Recognizing a dog with early CIPF is challenging

Funding Sources: H.P. Heikkilä-Laurila, Orion-Farmos Research Foundation, Finnish Veterinary Association, Finnish Veterinary Research Foundation, Finnish West Highland White Terrier, Breeding Club; M.M. Rajamäki, Finnish Veterinary Association, Finnish Veterinary Research Foundation.
Conflict of Interest: None.
Department of Equine and Small Animal Medicine, Faculty of Veterinary Medicine, University of Helsinki, PO Box 57 (Viikintie 49), Helsinki 00014, Finland
* Corresponding author.
E-mail address: henna.laurila@helsinki.fi

because the slowly progressive clinical signs can be confused with aging. Additionally, confirming CIPF requires very thorough examinations.

The first case series of CIPF in West Highland white terriers (WHWTs) was published in the late 1990s.[5] Reports of CIPF in other dog breeds (Staffordshire bull terrier, Schipperke, and Bull terrier) were described around the same time.[6,9] More recent studies of CIPF have aimed at defining the clinicopathologic findings of diseased WHWTs compared with controls matched by age and breed,[8] revealing histopathologic features,[7,10] findings detected on high-resolution CT (HRCT),[11] and assessing pulmonary hypertension (PHT) with Doppler.[12] Other studies include an investigation of surfactant protein (SP) C,[13] different potential fibrosis biomarkers,[14,15] and proteomic analysis of bronchoalveolar lavage (BAL) fluid (BALF) of WHWTs with CIPF.[16] Many questions regarding the disease remain unanswered. Cause and pathogenesis of the disease and the role of genetics are poorly understood and, therefore, are under active research.

DEFINITION AND HISTOPATHOLOGIC FEATURES

IPF belongs to a heterogenous group of ILDs that consist of several noninfectious and nonmalignant pulmonary diseases with overlapping clinicopathologic and radiographic features. ILDs affect the pulmonary interstitium, which is the space between the capillary endothelial and alveolar epithelial basement membranes.[17] In humans, more than 200 ILDs are recognized,[17] whereas far fewer ILDs are known to affect dogs.[18] In addition to CIPF, other described ILDs in dogs include diseases such as eosinophilic pneumonia, lymphocytic interstitial pneumonitis, bronchiolitis, obliterans with organizing pneumonia, endogenous lipid pneumonia, pulmonary alveolar proteinosis, silicosis, and asbestosis.[18] In humans, IPF belongs to an ILD subgroup named idiopathic interstitial pneumonias (IIPs). These are diseases of unknown causes resulting from damage to the pulmonary interstitium due to varying pattern of inflammation and fibrosis.[19] In dogs, such a subgroup and classification do not yet exist.

Currently, CIPF is probably the best-described canine ILD. It causes collagenous thickening of the pulmonary interstitium leading to impairment in the gas exchange.[7,8,10] Although CIPF is known to share clinical features with human IPF, the resemblance between the histopathologic pictures of human and canine disease was long in debate. Based on the recent (2013) study of Syrjä and colleagues,[10] CIPF seems to have histopathologic features of the two most common subtypes of human IIP, the usual interstitial pneumonia (UIP) and nonspecific interstitial pneumonia (NSIP). UIP is the histopathologic pattern of human IPF, and NSIP is the second most common IIP in humans and an important differential diagnosis for human IPF.[19]

CIPF is characterized histopathologically by two different patterns of interstitial fibrosis. All dogs appear to have mild-to-moderate, diffuse, mature fibrosis of the alveolar wall.[10] This pattern resembles the fibrosis pattern detected in human NSIP more than the patchy appearance of fibrosis in UIP. In addition to the mature fibrosis, most dogs have multifocal areas of fibrosis accentuation. In these areas, the fibrosis appears more severe, more cellular, and, therefore, less mature. This finding is more characteristic of human UIP than NSIP. In dogs, areas of fibrosis accentuation are either peribronchial or subpleural.[10] Honeycombing, profound alveolar epithelial changes, bronchial metaplasia of alveolar epithelium, and alveolar luminal changes, such as diffuse alveolar damage, can also be present in areas of more severe fibrosis. Fibroblast foci, very characteristic of human UIP, have not been found in dogs. Nevertheless, multifocal, scattered myofibroblasts have been detected in fibrotic interstitium. In addition to fibrosis, mild-to-moderate interstitial lymphoplasmacytic inflammation is present (**Figs. 1** and **2**).[10]

Histopathologic studies of CIPF have focused on describing the findings in WHWTs.[7,10] The only report of histopathologic features in breeds other than WHWTs was published by Lobetti and colleagues.[6] Whether there are differences in the histopathologic picture between WHWTs and other breeds is not yet clear.

CAUSE AND PATHOGENESIS

The causes of CIPF and IPF are currently unknown. In dogs, the strong predisposition of the WHWT to CIPF raises suspicion for a genetic background. In humans, familial and sporadic forms of IPF are recognized, with the familial form being less common.[1] However, family history of IPF was shown to be the strongest risk factor for human IPF in a recent study.[20] Other factors, such as environmental exposures,[20,21] cigarette smoking,[21,22] gastroesophageal reflux,[20,23] and possibly chronic viral infections,[24,25] have been recognized as potential risk factors for human IPF. Nevertheless, no unifying etiologic factor has been found.[26]

The pathogenetic mechanisms behind CIPF are not yet understood but are likely to be complex. Human IPF is hypothesized to arise from a chronic, repetitive, yet unknown insult to the distal lung parenchyma leading to injury and apoptosis of the alveolar epithelial cells. This is followed by an abnormal healing process, fibroblast and myofibroblast accumulation, and deposition of excess extracellular matrix, leading finally to the architectural changes seen in the IPF lung.[26–28] It is likely that IPF is the end result of a complicated dialogue between genetic and environmental factors.[20,29] This is also suspected in dogs although no epidemiologic studies have been performed.

Mutations in the SPs C and A2, and in the genes that maintain telomere length, have been associated with development of IPF in humans, but they explain only a small proportion of the population. Recent genetic studies suggest that mutations resulting in

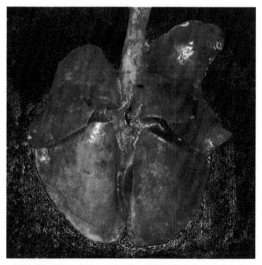

Fig. 1. Diffuse interstitial fibrosis of the lung in CIPF, with loss of pulmonary retraction and patchy multifocal accentuation of the lesions. (*Courtesy of* Pernilla Syrjä, DVM, Dipl ECVP, University of Helsinki, Finland.)

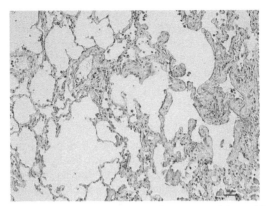

Fig. 2. The histopathology of CIPF in WHWTs is characterized by mild diffuse interstitial fibrosis (*left*) with multifocal areas of more severe interstitial fibrosis, alveolar epithelial atypia and hyperplasia, along with alveolar proteinosis and minimal interstitial inflammation (*right*). (*Courtesy of* Pernilla Syrjä, DVM, Dipl ECVP, University of Helsinki, Finland.)

defects in host defense and cell–cell adhesion could play an important role in IPF pathogenesis.[29,30] To date, only a single genetic study of CIPF has been published. After analyzing SP B and C in association with CIPF, Erikson and colleagues[13] (2009) found that SP C was absent in BALF from one of three dogs evaluated. In this dog, a mutation was detected at *SFTPC* exon 5.

As in humans, genetic factors could predispose a dog to development of disease, but other etiologic agents such as inhaled irritants are likely to be involved. Etiologic factors are difficult to trace because they may damage the lung for several years before CIPF is eventually diagnosed. Inbreeding of dogs, in this case WHWTs, offers a good resource to study these genetic mechanisms and their penetrance in CIPF.

SIGNALMENT AND CLINICAL SIGNS

CIPF usually affects middle-aged to older WHWTs. Occasionally, other terriers or other small breed dogs can be affected.[6,9,11,15,31] Human IPF more often affects males[1]; however, no sex predisposition has been reported in dogs. The usual age at the time of diagnosis varies from 8 to 15 years, but younger WHWTs with CIPF have also been reported.[5,12] Some of the non-WHWTs with CIPF have been substantially younger, with the youngest being only 3 years of age.[6] In humans, IPF typically manifests in the sixth and seventh decades and diagnosis in patients less than 50 years is rare.[1]

CIPF is considered an inevitably progressive disease. At the early phase of the disease affected dogs are probably quite normal. The mean duration of clinical signs when presented to the veterinarian has been estimated to be 8 to 13 months with great individual variation.[5,8,32] The most typical clinical signs are exercise intolerance and chronic cough in otherwise bright and alert dogs. Syncope, gagging, panting, and tachypnea are also reported. Not all affected dogs cough. Eventually, CIPF can cause respiratory difficulty, cyanosis, and respiratory failure.[5,8] Some dogs develop CIPF-related complications such as secondary respiratory tract infection or PHT. The authors are also aware of cases of pulmonary carcinoma in WHWTs with CIPF. In humans, an association exists between IPF and pulmonary carcinomas.[33] Pulmonary neoplasia coincident with IPF has also been reported in cats.[3]

In dogs with CIPF, mean survival time has been reported as 18 months from the beginning of clinical signs and less than 1 year from the time of diagnosis.[5] Nevertheless, survival time seems to vary greatly between individuals from some months to some years. Most human patients with IPF die within 5 years of diagnosis. However, several different progression patterns are recognized. In some patients, progression is slow whereas, in others, stable phases are interrupted by acute exacerbations. An accelerated variant of the disease also exists.[34] Whether these progression patterns also occur in dogs is currently not known.

DIAGNOSIS AND CLINICAL EXAMINATIONS

The diagnosis of CIPF is based on anamnestic information, findings in clinical examinations and diagnostic imaging, and exclusion of other respiratory diseases. Only histopathologic examination of lung tissue provides a definite diagnosis, but lung biopsies are seldom taken due to expense and the need for invasive surgery. The diagnosis if often confirmed at necropsy.

Dogs with CIPF are usually bright and alert due to adaptation to slowly developing respiratory impairment, but some severely affected dogs can be dyspneic and cyanotic. Bilateral, inspiratory Velcro crackles are a characteristic finding on lung auscultation,[5] but they might not be audible if the dog is breathing very shallowly.[8] In some dogs, crackles can even be heard without stethoscope when the dog is breathing with an open mouth. An abdominal breathing pattern is commonly present. A murmur, usually low-grade, right-sided, and systolic, can be heard in those dogs with tricuspid regurgitation due to PHT. Blood hematological and biochemical analyses do not show specific changes for CIPF but are commonly taken to rule out other reasons for exercise intolerance. The alkaline phosphatase concentration is frequently increased but, because such a change has also been found in healthy aged WHWTs, it is unlikely to be caused by hypoxemic liver damage.[8,32] Fecal examinations including the flotation and Baermann sedimentation methods are performed to rule out pulmonary parasites.

ARTERIAL OXYGENATION

Arterial blood gas analysis can be used to objectively estimate lung function. The method is easy to perform and gives a measurement of oxygenation capacity. It also provides an estimate of disease severity. Subsequent analyses can then be used to assess disease progression and possible treatment response. However, an arterial blood gas analysis cannot distinguish between lung function impairment due to fibrosis and inflammation. Measurement of hemoglobin saturation with oxygen by use of pulse oximetry is also used to estimate oxygenation. In the authors' opinion the pulse oximetry measurement can be misleading and offers at its best only an approximation of arterial oxygenation.

The sample for arterial blood gas analysis is drawn either from the femoral or the metatarsal artery into a heparinized syringe, any air bubbles are evacuated, and the sample is analyzed as soon as possible by a blood gas analyzer. The analysis provides measurements of PaO_2 and $PaCO_2$, and allows calculation of the alveolar-arterial oxygen gradient, $P(A-a)O_2$.[35]

Hypoxemia is a common finding in dogs with CIPF. In our previous study,[8] 90% of the WHWTs with CIPF were hypoxemic (PaO_2 less than 80 mm Hg[36]), and 45% had severe hypoxemia (PaO_2 less than 60 mm Hg[36]). Values for PaO_2, $PaCO_2$, and $P(A-a)O_2$ of WHWTs with CIPF and healthy control WHWTs are given in **Table 1**.

Table 1 Arterial blood gas analysis in WHWTs with CIPF (9 dogs) and healthy control WHWTs (11 dogs)		
	WHWTs with CIPF	Healthy WHWTs
PaO_2^a	65.5 ± 15.4 (33.5–87.4) mm Hg	99.1 ± 7.8 (89.6–113.0) mm Hg
$P(A-a)O_2^a$	50.1 ± 17.3 (28.0–84.7) mm Hg	17.5 ± 4.9 (10.7–26.8) mm Hg
$PaCO_2$	29.3 ± 3.8 (25.0–35.7) mm Hg	28.7 ± 3.8 (20.5–34.6) mm Hg

Results are given as mean ± SD and range.
[a] Statistically significant difference, $P<.001$.
Data from Heikkilä HP, Lappalainen AK, Day MJ, et al. Clinical, bronchoscopic, histopathologic, diagnostic imaging, and arterial oxygenation findings in West Highland white terriers with idiopathic pulmonary fibrosis. J Vet Intern Med 2011;25:433–9.

Despite such low oxygen levels, most of the dogs were bright, alert, and not in respiratory distress, indicating adaptation to a chronic, slowly progressing disease.

Hypoxemia resulting from IPF has a multifactorial background. In examinations on human IPF, only 20% of the hypoxemia was explained by alveolocapillary diffusion impairment due to thickened alveolocapillary membrane whereas the main reason for hypoxemia was ventilation–perfusion mismatch.[37]

DIAGNOSTIC IMAGING

Thoracic radiographs of dogs with CIPF commonly show a bronchointerstitial pattern, but only interstitial or predominantly bronchial patterns are also reported.[8,31,32] Usually radiographic changes are already moderate-to-severe when the animal is presented to the veterinarian (**Fig. 3**). Identifying early radiographic changes of CIPF can be problematic. Based on our previous study, healthy older WHWTs can also have mild bronchial or bronchointerstitial patterns in thoracic radiographs. Additionally, the thick skin typical for WHWTs can make the interpretation of subtle changes difficult.[8] Changes in thoracic radiographs are not sensitive or specific for CIPF.

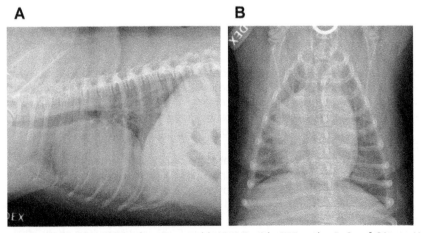

A   **B**

Fig. 3. Thoracic radiographs of a 12-year-old WHWT with CIPF and a PaO_2 of 64 mm Hg. Right lateral (A) and ventrodorsal (B) radiographs demonstrate a generalized bronchointerstitial lung pattern and large cardiac shadow. Extreme skin folds increase the overall opacity of the lungs. (*Courtesy of* Anu K. Lappalainen, DVM, PhD, University of Helsinki, Finland.)

Therefore, the main reason for taking them is to rule out other lung diseases such as neoplasia.

In dogs with CIPF, cardiac enlargement can be present in thoracic radiographs and is mainly caused by right-sided changes. This finding, together with lung densities and abnormal auscultation findings, sometimes results in false estimation of the presence of a primary heart disease. However, WHWT is not a breed typically affected by primary acquired heart diseases such as myxomatous mitral valve disease or cardiomyopathy. Therefore, an increased size of the heart shadow, especially in the dorsoventral view resulting in a reverse-D shaped cardiac silhouette and main pulmonary artery enlargement, should raise a suspicion of right-sided cardiac hypertrophy and possible presence of PHT. Further examination by Doppler echocardiography is required in these cases.[38] PHT is thought to result from an imbalance between pulmonary arterial vasoconstriction and vasodilatation, vascular remodeling due to an advanced lung disease, and chronic hypoxemia. Nevertheless, the pathogenesis of PHT is likely to be more complex than this and is not yet thoroughly understood.[39] PHT develops in a large number of WHWTs with CIPF. Schober and Baade[12] (2006) studied a group of WHWTs suffering from a chronic interstitial pulmonary disease with clinical signs and findings typical for CIPF. They estimated that PHT was a frequent finding affecting more than 40% of the WHWTs in their study. Similarly, PHT is very common in humans with IPF and is related to increased mortality.[39,40]

HRCT provides superior evaluation of the lung parenchyma compared with conventional thoracic radiographs. In human IPF, HRCT plays a crucial role in the diagnostic decision making and an HRCT diagnosis of IPF has a very high positive predictive value.[1] HRCT is also very useful in diagnosing CIPF.[8,11,32] Currently, the technique requires general anesthesia that might not be suitable for the most severely affected dogs due to increased anesthetic risk. The HRCT findings described in CIPF are ground glass opacity (a hazy increase in lung opacity), parenchymal bands, subpleural lines, subpleural interstitial thickening, peribronchovascular interstitial thickening, the interface sign, traction bronchiectasis, and honeycombing.[8,11,32] Consolidation can also occur[8,11] and, in some dogs, the bronchial walls can appear thickened.[32] Imaging findings in an individual dog are typically a combination of the above mentioned features (**Fig. 4**). The distribution of the lesions can be patchy[11] and the predilection site is reported to be the dorsocaudal lung lobes.[8] When attenuation of x-rays in lung tissue is evaluated quantitatively by measuring CT values, WHWTs with CIPF have significantly higher values than healthy WHWTs.[8]

In our previous study[8] and in the study of Johnson and colleagues[11] (2005), ground glass opacity was detected in all dogs with CIPF. The latter study suggested that honeycombing and traction bronchiectasis could be related to a more advanced CIPF; however, the authors have noticed that honeycombing and traction bronchiectasis can be present in dogs that lack severe hypoxemia. Honeycombing and traction bronchiectasis seem to be more common in human IPF, than in CIPF.

BRONCHOSCOPY AND BAL

Bronchoscopy and BAL provide useful information about the lung and airways. As for HRCT studies, the general condition and the severity of hypoxemia in the dog determine whether it is fit enough for the procedure. In the authors' experience, careful planning of anesthesia with supplemental oxygen before, during, and after bronchoscopy will make scoping possible even in severely hypoxemic dogs with CIPF.

Bronchoscopic findings detected in dogs with CIPF are nonspecific. Many dogs with CIPF seem to have some degree of bronchial involvement. It is not known

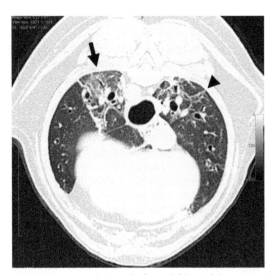

Fig. 4. A transverse HRCT image at the level of caudal lung lobes in an 11-year-old WHWT with CIPF and a PaO$_2$ of 57 mm Hg. Areas of ground glass opacity (*arrow*) and traction bronchiectasis (*arrowhead*) are seen dorsally. In this dog, the mean CT-value of all lung lobes was −709 HU, which is considerably higher than what is reported in healthy WHWTs. (*Courtesy of* Anu K. Lappalainen, DVM, PhD, University of Helsinki, Finland.)

whether this is an individual phenomenon or related to underlying CIPF. The presence of bronchoscopic changes cannot be used differentiate CIPF from chronic bronchitis (CB); however, bronchial changes such as hyperemia, mucus accumulation, and mucosal irregularities are usually more profound in CB than in CIPF.

Bronchoscopic changes reported in dogs with CIPF are tracheal collapse, bronchial mucosal irregularity, increased amount of bronchial mucus, bronchomalacia, dynamic airway collapse, and bronchiectasis.[8,32] Tracheal collapse and the increase in bronchial mucus are usually graded as mild-to moderate. Bronchial mucosal irregularity can at least partly be explained by age-related changes because it has also been detected in healthy, aged WHWTs and beagles.[8,41]

According to a survey of academic physicians, bronchoscopy is not commonly used in the diagnostic workup of human IPF.[42] The American Thoracic Society has provided clinical practice guidelines for BAL cellular analysis in ILDs only recently. Based on this, the usual BAL cell pattern in IPF is defined by increased macrophages and neutrophils, and mild-to-moderate eosinophilia can also be present. The lack of prominent lymphocytosis supports the diagnosis of IPF.[43]

In CIPF, BALF analysis usually shows an increase in the total cell count due to increased numbers of macrophages, neutrophils, and mast cells. In the differential cell counts, only a lower lymphocyte percentage was detected in dogs with CIPF compared with healthy dogs. Bacterial growth is not common.[8] A comparison of BALF analyses from WHWTs with CIPF with those obtained from healthy WHWTs is presented in **Table 2**.

TREATMENT

At the moment, there is no effective treatment of CIPF. Treatment is mainly used to reduce clinical signs on an individual basis and, secondly, to alleviate possible complications that can develop during the course of the disease. No clinical treatment

Table 2 BALF analysis in WHWTs with CIPF (11 dogs) and healthy control WHWTs (12 dogs)		
	WHWTs with CIPF	Healthy WHWTs
Total cell count (cells/μL)[a]	765, IQ 450–1120 (280–3115)	350, IQ 280–380 (265–420)
Macrophages (%)	84, IQ 66–88 (64–93)	78, IQ 76–82 (69–89)
Cells/μL[b]	672, IQ 304–1000 (178–2500)	269, IQ 225–289 (194–375)
Lymphocytes (%)[b]	6.4, IQ 4.4–13 (1.7–30)	16, IQ 14–19 (9.2–21)
Cells/μL	51, IQ 28–83 (14–335)	56, IQ 42–63 (39–79)
Neutrophils (%)	3.4, IQ 3.5–24 (3.0–30)	4.5, IQ 3.1–4.7 (0.9–6.2)
Cells/μL[a]	32, IQ 24–124 (10–753)	14, IQ 11–17 (2.8–18)
Eosinophils (%)	0.0, IQ 0.0–0.0 (0.0–2.0)	0.4, IQ 0.0–0.6 (0.0–2.0)
Cells/μL	0.0, IQ 0.0–1.8 (0.0–14)	1.5, IQ 0.0–1.8 (0.0–5.6)
Mast cells (%)	0.4, IQ 0.4–1.0 (0.0–2.5)	0.3, IQ 0.0–0.4 (0.0–0.9)
Cells/μL[b]	3.3, IQ 1.2–11 (0.0–64)	1.1, IQ 0.0–1.6 (0.0–3.2)

Results are given as median, interquartile range, and range.
[a] Statistically significant difference, $P<.01$.
[b] Statistically significant difference, $P<.05$.
Data from Heikkilä HP, Lappalainen AK, Day MJ, et al. Clinical, bronchoscopic, histopathologic, diagnostic imaging, and arterial oxygenation findings in West Highland white terriers with idiopathic pulmonary fibrosis. J Vet Intern Med 2011;25:433–9.

trials have been performed on dogs with CIPF and only anecdotal evidence exists for an effect of any drug. Expert opinions are based on recommendations for the treatment of human IPF as well as on the veterinarian's and owner's experience of treatment response.

Major effort has been put into finding novel medications for human IPF during the last decade. The developing knowledge about IPF pathogenesis has shifted treatment targets from inflammation toward the aberrant wound healing process. Several studies have investigated the use of immunomodulatory therapies, anticoagulant agents, endothelin receptor antagonists, vasodilators, antifibrotics, and cytokine inhibitors, without success.[44] The use of corticosteroids was found to be of no benefit, and a standard-of-care combination therapy with prednisone, azathioprine, and N-acetylcysteine was revealed to be harmful in a recent study.[45] This is no longer recommended for treatment of human IPF; however, a trial on N-acetylcysteine monotherapy is ongoing. In pilot studies, this antioxidant precursor has shown potential beneficial effects, but there is not yet enough data to support its use. At the moment, there is no treatment that can reverse the chronic fibrotic changes of human IPF. Lung transplantation is the only therapeutic modality known to increase survival.[44]

A major turning point was reached when pirfenidone was approved for the clinical treatment of human IPF in Asia and Europe. Pirfenidone has well-established antifibrotic, antioxidant, and antiinflammatory effects in experimental rodent models of fibrosis.[28] In Japanese studies on human patients with IPF, pirfenidone slowed the decline in lung function. Due to concerns related to the lack of survival benefit, more clinical studies are currently underway to further clarify its effect.[44] Pirfenidone could possibly be considered for treatment of CIPF. Although the pharmacokinetics of pirfenidone have been studied in dogs,[46] the safety of the drug in dogs is not known and there are no published reports of its clinical use in dogs.

Corticosteroids are used in the treatment of humans with NSIP. Patients with the cellular variant of NSIP have a better treatment response and prognosis than those with IPF.[19] Based on the potential benefit of corticosteroids in human NSIP and because many dogs have concurrent bronchial changes, oral corticosteroids might have a role in the treatment of CIPF. Corcoran and colleagues[5] (1999) reported previously that some dogs with CIPF seem to respond to corticosteroid treatment. Based also on the authors' experience, corticosteroids seem to alleviate cough in many dogs although no clear effect on arterial oxygenation is detected. Because the combination of a high dose of corticosteroids and azathioprine was shown to be potentially deleterious in humans with IPF,[47] this combination should probably not be used in dogs either.

In CIPF, antitussives can be used if cough is irritating. Bronchodilators such as theophylline may be tried. Theophylline causes mild bronchodilatation, enhances mucociliary clearance, and increases contractibility of the diaphragmatic muscle.[48] Combination therapy with theophylline and corticosteroids has previously been recommended for treatment of CIPF.[5] Theophylline should be administrated with caution in hypoxemic animals and in combination with various drugs, including enrofloxacin and corticosteroids.[49]

Dogs with CIPF can experience worsening of respiratory function during the course of the disease. The cause for worsening should be diagnosed, if possible, and treated accordingly. Pneumonia should be suspected if leukocytosis or a left shift is detected together with newly developed alveolar density in thoracic radiographs. Unfortunately, the reason for the acute worsening is not always found. In humans with IPF, an unexpected, accelerated phase of lung function decline in the absence of any causative factor is called an acute exacerbation of IPF. Despite intensive care and empiric treatment with high doses of corticosteroids, cytotoxic agents, broad-spectrum antibiotics, and mechanical ventilation, the mortality of acute exacerbation in IPF approaches 50%.[47]

Usually, treatment of PHT is focused on treating the underlying disease. Because no efficacious treatment exists for CIPF, treatment is directly targeted to reduce pulmonary arterial pressure.[38] Studies on the treatment of PHT in dogs are scarce, but use of sildenafil, a phosphodiesterase-5 inhibitor, has been evaluated.[50,51] There is a theoretical concern that hypoxemia could worsen with PHT treatment because selective pulmonary arterial vasodilatation caused by medication could potentially increase ventilation perfusion mismatch.[39] However, the official statement for human IPF management notes that patients with moderate-to-severe PHT might benefit from PHT treatment.[1] The authors' have experienced that treatment with sildenafil can improve exercise tolerance in dogs with CIPF and PHT, and dogs appear brighter and more alert after starting treatment. The authors use a starting dose of approximately 1 mg/kg by mouth three times a day.

Treatment with proton pump inhibitors or histamine-2 receptor blockers could be considered if corticosteroid therapy is started because hypoxemia can make the dog more prone to adverse gastrointestinal effects. In human patients with IPF, gastroesophageal reflux, either symptomatic or occult, is very common, and microaspiration is speculated to have a role in the pathogenesis of IPF.[23,52] It is currently unknown whether gastroesophageal reflux is as prevalent in dogs with IPF.

BIOMARKERS

Diagnosing CIPF requires laborious examinations and can be challenging, especially when differentiating it from the main differential diagnosis, CB. CB carries a better prognosis and responds better to treatment. Both CIPF and CB can cause cough and exercise intolerance, and diseased dogs are usually of similar age and are small breed dogs.[15,48] There are no specific findings in thoracic radiographs for either of the diseases, and differentiation with bronchoscopy is not possible because bronchial changes can be encountered in both. Reaching the CIPF diagnosis can require HRCT, which is expensive and not always applicable, or histologic investigation of the lung tissue. Identification of a noninvasive, measurable biomarker of fibrosis could help with the diagnosis.

A good biomarker is sensitive, specific, cost-effective, and practical to use.[53] In CIPF, search for suitable biomarkers is ongoing and some potential markers have already been found. Procollagen type III amino terminal propeptide (PIINP) is a marker of fibroblast activity and enhanced collagen turnover. PIIINP levels are elevated in humans with IPF. In dogs with CIPF, PIIINP levels are elevated in BALF and can be used to differentiate CIPF from CB with reasonable accuracy. However, serum PIIINP concentrations cannot distinguish between different chronic lung diseases. Although BALF biomarker probably better represents the production of collagen in the lungs and is less influenced by other factors than serum markers, its use is less practical.[15]

Endothelin-1 (ET-1) is a vasoactive, proinflammatory, and profibrotic peptide that is elevated in humans with IPF, both in serum and BALF. Serum ET-1 is also significantly elevated in dogs with CIPF compared with dogs with eosinophilic bronchopneumopathy, healthy dogs, or dogs with CB. ET-1 could be useful in diagnosing CIPF and differentiating it from other lung diseases. A clear advantage is that it can be measured from serum.[14]

Proteomics has also been used to examine a large scale of expressed proteins in BALF to find those specific for CIPF. Lilja-Maula and colleagues[16] (2013) performed a gel-based quantitative two-dimensional differential gel electrophoresis proteomic study followed by mass spectrometry in WHWTs with CIPF. Unfortunately, comparison of BALF proteomes between healthy dogs and dogs with CIPF or CB revealed no CIPF-specific proteins. Results showed similar changes in CIPF and CB groups, suggesting a common response to disease in otherwise different lung diseases.

In addition to using biomarkers in diagnostics, biomarker research could better define the pathogenesis of CIPF in dogs. Further studies using combinations of biomarkers could clarify the disease process in CIPF and help define the course of the disease in dogs. It is hoped that, in the near future, a biomarker that differentiates WHWTs that will later develop CIPF from those that will not could even be used in selecting dogs for breeding.

REFERENCES

1. Raghu G, Collard HR, Egan JJ, et al. An official ATS/ERS/JRS/ALAT statement: idiopathic pulmonary fibrosis: evidence-based guidelines for diagnosis and management. Am J Respir Crit Care Med 2011;183(6):788–824.
2. Liebow AA. Definition and classification of interstitial pneumonias in human pathology. Prog Respir Res 1975;8(1):21–31.
3. Cohn LA, Norris CR, Hawkins EC, et al. Identification and characterization of an idiopathic pulmonary fibrosis-like condition in cats. J Vet Intern Med 2004;18(5):632–41.
4. Williams K, Malarkey D, Cohn L, et al. Identification of spontaneous feline idiopathic pulmonary fibrosis: morphology and ultrastructural evidence for a type II pneumocyte defect. Chest 2004;125(6):2278–88.
5. Corcoran BM, Cobb M, Martin MW, et al. Chronic pulmonary disease in West Highland white terriers. Vet Rec 1999;144(22):611–6.
6. Lobetti RG, Milner R, Lane E. Chronic idiopathic pulmonary fibrosis in five dogs. J Am Anim Hosp Assoc 2001;37(2):119–27.

7. Norris AJ, Naydan DK, Wilson DW. Interstitial lung disease in West Highland White Terriers. Vet Pathol 2005;42(1):35–41.

8. Heikkilä HP, Lappalainen AK, Day MJ, et al. Clinical, bronchoscopic, histopathologic, diagnostic imaging, and arterial oxygenation findings in West Highland white terriers with idiopathic pulmonary fibrosis. J Vet Intern Med 2011;25(3): 433–9.

9. Corcoran BM, Dukes-McEwan J, Rhind S, et al. Idiopathic pulmonary fibrosis in a Staffordshire bull terrier with hypothyroidism. J Small Anim Pract 1999;40(4): 185–8.

10. Syrjä P, Heikkilä HP, Rönty M, et al. The histopathology of idiopathic pulmonary fibrosis in West Highland white terriers shares features of both nonspecific interstitial pneumonia and usual interstitial pneumonia in man. J Comp Pathol 2013; 149:303–13.

11. Johnson VS, Corcoran BM, Wotton PR, et al. Thoracic high-resolution computed tomographic findings in dogs with canine idiopathic pulmonary fibrosis. J Small Anim Pract 2005;46(8):381–8.

12. Schober KE, Baade H. Doppler echocardiographic prediction of pulmonary hypertension in West Highland white terriers with chronic pulmonary disease. J Vet Intern Med 2006;20(4):912–20.

13. Erikson M, von Euler H, Ekman E, et al. Surfactant protein C in canine pulmonary fibrosis. J Vet Intern Med 2009;23:1170–4.

14. Krafft E, Heikkilä H, Jespers P, et al. Serum and bronchoalveolar lavage fluid endothelin-1 concentrations as diagnostic biomarkers of canine idiopathic pulmonary fibrosis. J Vet Intern Med 2011;25:990–6.

15. Heikkilä HP, Krafft E, Jespers P, et al. Procollagen type III amino terminal propeptide concentrations in dogs with idiopathic pulmonary fibrosis compared with chronic bronchitis and eosinophilic bronchopneumopathy. Vet J 2013; 196:52–6.

16. Lilja-Maula LI, Palviainen MJ, Heikkilä HP, et al. Proteomic analysis of bronchoalveolar lavage fluid samples obtained from West Highland White Terriers with idiopathic pulmonary fibrosis, dogs with chronic bronchitis, and healthy dogs. Am J Vet Res 2013;74(1):148–54.

17. Cushley M, Davison A, du Bois R, et al. The diagnosis, assessment and treatment of diffuse parenchymal lung disease in adults. Thorax 1999;54:S1–30.

18. Reinero CR, Cohn LA. Interstitial lung diseases. Vet Clin North Am Small Anim Pract 2007;37(5):937–47.

19. American Thoracic Society, European Respiratory Society. American Thoracic Society, European Respiratory Society. International multidisciplinary consensus classification of the idiopathic interstitial pneumonias. Am J Respir Crit Care Med 2002;165(2):277–304.

20. García-Sancho C, Buendía-Roldán I, Fernández-Plata MR, et al. Familial pulmonary fibrosis is the strongest risk factor for idiopathic pulmonary fibrosis. Respir Med 2011;105(12):1902–7.

21. Taskar VS, Coultas DB. Is idiopathic pulmonary fibrosis an environmental disease? Proc Am Thorac Soc 2006;3(4):293–8.

22. Baumgartner KB, Samet JM, Stidley CA, et al. Cigarette smoking: a risk factor for idiopathic pulmonary fibrosis. Am J Respir Crit Care Med 1997;155(1): 242–8.

23. Gribbin J, Hubbard R, Smith C. Role of diabetes mellitus and gastrooesophageal reflux in the aetiology of idiopathic pulmonary fibrosis. Respir Med 2009;103(6):927–31.

24. Tang YW, Johnson JE, Browning PJ, et al. Herpesvirus DNA is consistently detected in lungs of patients with idiopathic pulmonary fibrosis. J Clin Microbiol 2003;41(6):2633–40.
25. Calabrese F, Kipar A, Lunardi F, et al. Herpes virus infection is associated with vascular remodeling and pulmonary hypertension in idiopathic pulmonary fibrosis. PLoS One 2013;8(2):e55715.
26. Kottmann RM, Hogan CH, Phipps RP, et al. Determinants of initiation and progression of idiopathic pulmonary fibrosis. Respirology 2009;14:917–33.
27. Harari S, Caminati A. IPF: new insight on pathogenesis and treatment. Allergy 2010;65(5):537–53.
28. Loomis-King H, Flaherty KR, Moore BB. Pathogenesis, current treatments and future directions for idiopathic pulmonary fibrosis. Curr Opin Pharmacol 2013; 13(3):377–85.
29. Fingerlin TE, Murphy E, Zhang W, et al. Genome-wide association study identifies multiple susceptibility loci for pulmonary fibrosis. Nat Genet 2013;45:613–20.
30. Seibold MA, Wise AL, Speer MC, et al. A common MUC5B promoter polymorphism and pulmonary fibrosis. N Engl J Med 2011;364(16):1503–12.
31. Webb JA, Armstrong J. Chronic idiopathic pulmonary fibrosis in a West Highland white terrier. Can Vet J 2002;43(9):703–5.
32. Corcoran BM, King LG, Schwarz T, et al. Further characterisation of the clinical features of chronic pulmonary disease in West Highland white terriers. Vet Rec 2011;168:355.
33. Aubry MC, Myers JL, Douglas WW, et al. Primary pulmonary carcinoma in patients with idiopathic pulmonary fibrosis. Mayo Clin Proc 2002;77(8):763–70.
34. Selman M, Carrillo G, Estrada A, et al. Accelerated variant of idiopathic pulmonary fibrosis: clinical behavior and gene expression pattern. PLoS One 2007; 2(5):e482–6.
35. Day TK. Blood gas analysis. Vet Clin North Am Small Anim Pract 2002;32(5): 1031–48.
36. Haskins SC. Interpretation of blood gas measurements. In: King LG, editor. Textbook of respiratory disease in dogs and cats. St Louis (MO): Saunders Elsevier; 2004. p. 181–93.
37. Erbes R, Schaberg T, Loddenkemper R. Lung function tests in patients with idiopathic pulmonary fibrosis. Chest 1997;111(1):51–7.
38. Campbell FE. Cardiac effects of pulmonary disease. Vet Clin North Am Small Anim Pract 2007;37(5):949–62.
39. Smith JS, Gorbett D, Mueller J, et al. Pulmonary hypertension and idiopathic pulmonary fibrosis—a dastardly duo. Am J Med Sci 2013;346:221–5.
40. Frankel SK, Schwarz MI. Update in idiopathic pulmonary fibrosis. Curr Opin Pulm Med 2009;15(5):463–9.
41. Mercier E, Bolognin M, Hoffmann AC, et al. Influence of age on bronchoscopic findings in healthy beagle dogs. Vet J 2011;187:225–8.
42. Collard HR, Loyd JE, King TE Jr, et al. Current diagnosis and management of idiopathic pulmonary fibrosis: a survey of academic physicians. Respir Med 2007;101(9):2011.
43. Meyer KC, Raghu G, Baughman RP, et al. An official American Thoracic Society clinical practice guideline: the clinical utility of bronchoalveolar lavage cellular analysis in interstitial lung disease. Am J Respir Crit Care Med 2012;185(9): 1004–14.
44. Rafii R, Juarez MM, Albertson TE, et al. A review of current and novel therapies for idiopathic pulmonary fibrosis. J Thorac Dis 2013;5(1):48–73.

45. Raghu G, Anstrom KJ, King TE Jr, et al. Prednisone, azathioprine, and N-acetyl-cysteine for pulmonary fibrosis. N Engl J Med 2012;366(21):1968–77.

46. Bruss ML, Margolin SB, Giri SN. Pharmacokinetics of orally administered pirfenidone in male and female beagles. J Vet Pharmacol Ther 2004;27(5):361–7.

47. Adamali HI, Maher TM. Current and novel drug therapies for idiopathic pulmonary fibrosis. Drug Des Devel Ther 2012;6:261–71.

48. Kuehn NF. Chronic bronchitis in dogs. In: King LG, editor. Textbook of respiratory disease in dogs and cats. St Louis (MO): Saunders; 2004. p. 379–87.

49. Plumb DC. Plumb's veterinary drug handbook. 7th edition. Ames (IA): Wiley-Blackwell; 2011.

50. Kellum HB, Stepien RL. Sildenafil citrate therapy in 22 dogs with pulmonary hypertension. J Vet Intern Med 2007;21(6):1258–64.

51. Brown AJ, Davison E, Sleeper MM. Clinical efficacy of sildenafil in treatment of pulmonary arterial hypertension in dogs. J Vet Intern Med 2010;24(4):850–4.

52. Raghu G, Freudenberger T, Yang S, et al. High prevalence of abnormal acid gastro-oesophageal reflux in idiopathic pulmonary fibrosis. Eur Respir J 2006; 27(1):136–42.

53. Louhelainen N, Myllärniemi M, Rahman I, et al. Airway biomarkers of the oxidant burden in asthma and chronic obstructive pulmonary disease: current and future perspectives. Int J Chron Obstruct Pulmon Dis 2008;3(4):585–602.

Bacterial Pneumonia in Dogs and Cats

Jonathan D. Dear, DVM

KEYWORDS

- Bacterial pneumonia • Lower respiratory tract infection • Canine • Feline
- Lower airway disease

KEY POINTS

- Bacterial pneumonia is recognized much more commonly in dogs than in cats.
- Viral infection followed by bacterial invasion is common in young dogs, whereas aspiration pneumonia and foreign body pneumonia seem to be more common in older dogs.
- Clinical signs can be acute or chronic and do not always reflect a primary respiratory condition.
- Definitive diagnosis requires detection of intracellular bacteria in airway cytology or clinically significant bacterial growth from an airway sample, although relevant clinical findings are often used.
- Treatment requires identification of underlying diseases associated with pneumonia, appropriate antibiotic therapy, and control of airway secretions.

INTRODUCTION

Bacterial pneumonia remains one of the most common clinical diagnoses in dogs with either acute or chronic respiratory disease. New research suggests a complex relationship between viral respiratory diseases and development of bacterial pneumonia in dogs. Over the past decade, much has been discovered about the convoluted interplay between host and environmental factors that leads to this complex of diseases. In cats, bacterial pneumonia is less commonly identified than inflammatory feline bronchial disease.

CLASSIFICATION OF BACTERIAL PNEUMONIA
Aspiration

Aspiration pneumonia results from the inadvertent inhalation of gastric acid and/or ingesta and remains a common cause of bacterial pneumonia, accounting for roughly 23% of clinical diagnoses in a study of human patients admitted to the intensive care

Disclosures: None.
William R. Pritchard Veterinary Medical Teaching Hospital, University of California–Davis, One Shields Avenue, Davis, CA 95616, USA
E-mail address: jddear@ucdavis.edu

unit.[1] Although inhalation of gastroesophageal material is a common theme, different factors lead to the development of this phenomenon. Risk factors that have been identified for the development of aspiration pneumonia include esophageal disease, refractory vomiting, seizures, prolonged anesthesia, and laryngeal dysfunction (**Table 1**).[2]

In a healthy animal, physiologic and anatomic features reduce the chance of aspiration. During a normal swallow, fluid and food are propelled caudally in the oropharynx and through the upper esophageal sphincter by contraction of the oral cavity and tongue. At the same time, the epiglottis retracts to cover the laryngeal aditus and protect the trachea from particulate inhalation. Adduction of the arytenoid cartilages then contributes to further occlusion of the upper airways. Any process impeding these primary defenses or inhibiting the normal swallowing reflexes increases the likelihood of aspiration.

Aspiration injury results from inhalation of either sterile, acidic gastric contents (resulting from vomiting or gastric regurgitation) or of septic material from gastric or oral secretions. Irritation induced by acid inhalation promotes a local environment in which bacterial colonization can develop and lead to bacterial pneumonia. The severity of disease varies depending on the quantity and nature of the material aspirated as well as the length of time between the event and its diagnosis. Conscious patients with intact airway reflexes tend to cough and prevent massive aspiration injury. Animals under anesthesia or with reduced airway reflexes because of neurologic disorders are less likely to cough in response to the aspiration event and are, therefore, more likely to develop diffuse pulmonary infiltrates and acute lung injury. In many instances aspiration injuries occur under general anesthesia and the presence of a cuffed endotracheal tube does not prevent inadvertent aspiration.

Canine Infectious Pneumonia

Infectious, or community–acquired, pneumonias in dogs commonly begin with viral colonization and infection of the upper respiratory tract (canine respiratory coronavirus, herpesvirus, pneumovirus, and parainfluenza virus, among others).[3] Often, such diseases are acute and self-limiting, but in a subset of dogs inflammation associated

Table 1 **Factors associated with aspiration pneumonia**	
Gastrointestinal disease • Refractory vomiting caused by systemic or metabolic disease • Pancreatitis • Intussusception • Foreign body obstruction • Ileus	Anesthesia • Prolonged anesthesia • Postprocedural upper airway obstruction
Esophageal disease • Megaesophagus • Esophageal motility disorder • Hiatal hernia • Esophageal stricture • Esophagitis	Neurologic disease • Polyneuropathy • Myasthenia gravis • Seizure • Conditions leading to prolonged recumbency
Cricopharyngeal dyssynchrony Muscular dystrophy Oropharyngeal dysphagia Laryngeal disease	Breed • Bulldog • Golden retriever • Pug • Cocker spaniel • English springer spaniel

Data from Refs.[11,21,22]; with permission.

with these organisms immobilizes the host's immune defenses and predisposes infection with other (often bacterial) respiratory pathogens.[4] Many bacteria have been implicated in canine infectious respiratory disease (CIRD), although special focus has been directed toward *Streptococcus* (specifically *Streptococcus equi* subsp *zooepidemicus* and *S canis*), *Mycoplasma cynos*, and *Bordetella bronchiseptica*.

CIRD is especially prevalent in dogs naive to the pathogens and exposed in overcrowded, stressful environments such as animal shelters, boarding kennels, and treatment facilities. The pathophysiology associated with this disease and infectious lower respiratory tract disease in cats is discussed later in this article (**Boxes 1 and 2**).

Foreign Body

Inhaled foreign bodies carry mixed bacterial and fungal organisms into the lung and are associated with focal pneumonias that are often initially responsive to antimicrobial medications but relapse shortly after discontinuation of therapy.[5,6] Foreign bodies reported in the veterinary literature include grass awns, plant materials, or plastic materials.[6] Organisms associated with grass awn inhalation include *Pasteurella*, *Streptococcus*, *Nocardia*, *Actinomyces*, and anaerobic bacteria.[6,7] Most often, foreign material remains at the carina or enters caudodorsal principal bronchi (accessory, right and left caudal lobar bronchi).

Features associated with pulmonary foreign bodies include:

- Young, sporting breeds
- Environmental exposure to grass awns
- Focal, recurrent radiographic alveolar pattern
- History of other cutaneous or visceral foreign bodies
- Spontaneous pneumothorax or pyothorax

Box 1
CIRD complex: changing the nature of kennel cough

CIRD complex (formerly known as kennel cough) is a syndrome in which multiple pathogens, both viral and bacterial, coinfect either naive, immunocompromised dogs or previously vaccinated dogs. This complex is multifactorial and it is likely that both host and environmental factors play a role in the development of illness.[27] Organisms associated with this disease are ubiquitous, especially in overcrowded housing facilities such as animal shelters and training facilities. It is likely that stress induced by the new environment and exposure to novel pathogens both play a role in development of disease.

In most cases, respiratory signs are present for days to weeks and most animals show mild to moderate clinical signs. Viral infections typically cause either a bronchopneumonia or bronchointerstitial pneumonia because of their propensity to infect and damage type I pneumocytes.[28] As the condition progresses, desquamation of the respiratory epithelium and aggregation of inflammatory cells further reduce the lungs' natural defenses, increasing the potential for secondary bacterial colonization and infection.

Previous studies have implicated viral organisms such as canine adenovirus or canine parainfluenza[29] as major participants in CIRD, although recent studies have proposed novel respiratory pathogens such as canine respiratory coronavirus,[3,20,30,31] canine influenza virus,[20] and canine herpesvirus[32] as additional important pathogens associated with CIRD. *B bronchiseptica*,[33] *Streptococcus canis*, *S equi* subsp *zooepidemicus*,[29] and *M cynos*[3,34] have been implicated as secondary bacterial infections associated with CIRD. *S equi* subsp *zooepidemicus* infections, in particular, have been associated with a rapidly progressive and often fatal hemorrhagic pneumonia.[27,35] Some strains identified in outbreaks of this pathogen have been identified as resistant to tetracycline antibiotics, which are often the drug of choice prescribed for other bacterial pathogens associated with this complex.

Box 2
Feline lower respiratory tract infections

Organisms that have been reported as lower respiratory pathogens of cats include *Pasteurella* spp, *Escherichia coli*, *Staphylococcus* spp, *Streptococcus* spp, *Pseudomonas* spp, *B bronchiseptica*, and *Mycoplasma* spp,[36] and specific attention has been paid to *Mycoplasma* spp because of a possible association with the induction and exacerbation of asthma in adult and pediatric human patients.[37] However, the association between lower respiratory infection and chronic inflammatory lower airway disease in cats is unclear and is a topic of ongoing interest.

Mycoplasma species are considered normal flora in the upper respiratory tract and their role is controversial in lower respiratory tract infection. Because they are rarely identified cytologically, and specific culture or polymerase chain reaction is needed to document the presence of these organisms, the role of *Mycoplasma* in cats (as well as in dogs) remains difficult to define.

Normal thoracic radiographs do not rule out the possibility of an airway foreign body[8] and even computed tomography (CT) can fail to identify an affected bronchus. Chronic pulmonary foreign bodies are associated with marked inflammation that can lead to massive airway remodeling and bronchiectasis that, when seen on radiographs, should raise the degree of suspicion for foreign body.[5]

Nosocomial

Ventilator-associated pneumonia (VAP) is a common cause of hospital-acquired pneumonia in people, although there are few veterinary reports in the literature. Colonization of the oropharynx by pathogenic and multidrug-resistant bacteria occurs and the endotracheal tube acts as a conduit to transmit pathogens into the airways, which leads to tracheobronchitis and potentially pneumonia. In addition, any animal with a compromised respiratory tract or serious systemic disease is particularly prone to development of infectious airway disease while hospitalized.

The use of mechanical ventilation in human patients raises the risk of nosocomial infection by 6-fold to 20-fold.[9] No published studies assess the risk in ventilated veterinary patients, although a study investigating differences in bacterial sensitivity between ventilated and nonventilated patients suggested that patients requiring mechanical ventilation were more likely to be infected with bacteria resistant to the antimicrobials most commonly used in veterinary practice.[8] This finding parallels the increase in incidence of multidrug-resistant VAP in human medicine.[9]

Immune Dysfunction

Both the innate and adaptive immune systems protect against the development of infectious airway disease, and a breakdown in either increases the likelihood of opportunistic infection (**Table 2**). Congenital immunodeficiencies have been recognized that make an animal particularly sensitive to infectious disease. Young animals are especially prone to the development of bacterial pneumonia because of their naive immune systems, and when coupled with alterations to the innate immune system, such as primary ciliary dyskinesia (PCD) or complement deficiency, the risk of life-threatening infection increases greatly (see *Veterinary Clinics of North America* 2007;37(5):845–60 for a comprehensive review of respiratory defenses in health and disease).

Any cause of systemic immunocompromise increases the risk for bacterial pneumonia, and any additional alterations to the body's natural defense mechanisms increase the risk. Medications such as chemotherapy, immunosuppressive therapy, or antitussive therapy significantly increase the likelihood of bacterial pneumonia.

Table 2		
Conditions leading to impaired immune function and resulting in increased risk of pneumonia		
	Congenital	Acquired
Innate	Primary ciliary dyskinesia	Bronchiectasis
	Complement deficiency	Secondary ciliary dyskinesia
	Leukocyte adhesion deficiency	
Adaptive	Immunoglobulin deficiency	Retrovirus infection (eg, FIV, FeLV)
	Severe combined immunodeficiency	Endocrine or metabolic disease (eg, DM or HAC)
		Chemotherapy and other immunosuppressive therapy
		Splenectomy

Abbreviations: DM, diabetes mellitus; FeLV, feline leukemia virus; FIV, feline immunodeficiency virus; HAC, hyperadrenocorticism.
Data from Refs.[23–25]; with permission.

Underlying respiratory viruses or systemic viruses such as feline leukemia virus and feline immunodeficiency virus have the potential to enhance the severity of respiratory illness.

CLINICAL SIGNS

Clinical signs of bacterial pneumonia vary depending on its cause, severity, and chronicity of disease. They can be acute or peracute in onset or can display an insidious onset, resulting in chronic illness. Early in disease, mild signs such as an intermittent, soft cough might be the only evidence of disease. As infection spreads, clinical signs worsen and often include a refractory, productive cough, exercise intolerance, anorexia, and severe lethargy. Owners can note a change in the respiratory pattern, with increased panting or rapid breathing and, in cases of severe infection, cyanosis and orthopnea can be observed. In general, these systemic signs are more obviously displayed in dogs than in cats.

Cats with pneumonia can display similar clinical signs, although the cough can be misinterpreted as a wretch or vomit by owners. Clinical signs and radiographic findings can also be considered consistent with inflammatory airway disease. As disease worsens, cats can become tachypneic with short, shallow breaths and nasal flaring.[10] Owners rarely notice exercise intolerance associated with bacterial pneumonia.

PHYSICAL EXAMINATION

As with the history and clinical signs of bacterial pneumonia, physical examination findings vary with the state and severity of disease. Dogs or cats with mild disease can have no abnormalities detected on physical examination. An early clue to the diagnosis might be a change in the respiratory pattern, with an increase in rate and effort. The clinician needs to pay close attention to thoracic auscultation because adventitious lung sounds (crackles and wheezes) can be subtle, focal, or intermittent. In many cases, only harsh or increased lung sounds are detected rather than crackles.[5] The examination should also include a thorough auscultation of the trachea and upper airway for evidence of upper airway signs (eg, nasal congestion or discharge) that can result from lower airway infection, either as an extension of epithelial infection or from nasopharyngeal regurgitation of lower airway secretions.

Animals with bacterial pneumonia generally present with mixed inspiratory and expiratory signs, similar to those seen with other diseases of the pulmonary parenchyma. Fever is detected in 16% to 50% of cases, so it is not a reliable indicator of disease.[4,11–13]

DIAGNOSIS

Bacterial pneumonia implies sepsis of the lower airway and lungs, so the diagnosis is confirmed by showing septic suppurative inflammation on airway cytology obtained through bronchoalveolar lavage (BAL) or tracheal wash, along with a positive microbiology culture. In some cases, this is completed easily and yields results consistent with clinical suspicion. However, financial limitations or patient concerns can inhibit the ability to collect samples needed to document specifically a bacterial infection, and in those cases a clinical diagnosis of bacterial pneumonia might be presumed based on available information.

A clinical diagnosis of bacterial pneumonia should be reached after obtaining compelling evidence to suggest a bacterial cause for the animal's clinical signs (after excluding other causes), with appropriate resolution of signs following suitable antimicrobial therapy. Acute bacterial pneumonia is a common diagnosis in the small animal clinic and can often be easily identified; however, early and chronic pneumonias are more challenging to recognize because clinical signs can be subtle.

Hematology

The complete blood count is a useful diagnostic test in animals with respiratory signs. Bacterial pneumonias are typically associated with an inflammatory leukogram, characterized primarily by a neutrophilia, with or without a left shift and variable evidence of toxic changes,[7,14] although the absence of inflammatory change does not exclude the possibility of pneumonia.[4,11] Furthermore, the leukogram and differential can provide clues to suggest that bacterial pneumonia is less likely. For example, eosinophilia in an animal with respiratory signs would suggest eosinophilic bronchopneumopathy or parasitic lung diseases as an underlying cause rather than a bacterial cause. The erythrogram and platelet evaluation are generally not helpful in determining a bacterial cause of respiratory disease.

A biochemistry panel, urinalysis, and fecal flotation do not always contribute to the diagnosis of bacterial pneumonia but can provide clues to the presence of metabolic or endocrine diseases that could make the development of bacterial pneumonia more likely.

Thoracic Radiography

Thoracic radiographs are crucial diagnostic tests in the evaluation of lower airway and pulmonary parenchymal disease. Radiographic evidence of bacterial pneumonia can appear as a focal, multifocal, or diffuse alveolar pattern, although early in the disease process infiltrates might be primarily interstitial (**Figs. 1** and **2**). Ventral lung lobes are most commonly affected in aspiration pneumonia, and a caudodorsal pattern is expected with inhaled foreign bodies or hematogenous bacterial spread. A lobar sign can be seen in cases of aspiration pneumonia in which the right middle lung lobe is most often affected (**Table 3**).

Three-view thoracic radiographs (left lateral, right lateral, and either dorsoventral or ventrodorsal views) should be obtained when screening for pneumonia because differential aeration associated with positional atelectasis can either mask or highlight pulmonary changes. For example, a radiograph taken in left lateral recumbency is preferred when aspiration is suspected because it increases aeration of the right middle lung lobe, the most commonly affected lobe.

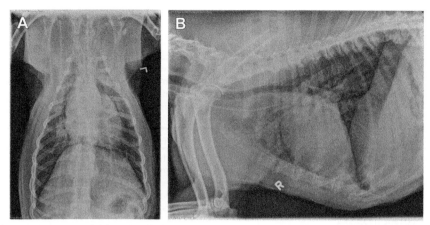

Fig. 1. Dorsoventral (*A*) and right lateral (*B*) thoracic radiographs from a dog with an alveolar pattern in the cranioventral lung lobes, suggesting aspiration. In this case, the left cranial lobes were most affected which are most easily examined on the right lateral view. In many cases the right middle lung lobe is most affected, necessitating a left lateral orthogonal view.

Diffuse radiographic involvement is expected to suggest more severe disease, although radiographic changes lag behind clinical disease. Consequently, bacterial pneumonia cannot be ruled out in patients with acute onset of clinical signs and unremarkable radiographs.[7]

Advanced Imaging

Advanced imaging is rarely necessary in the diagnosis of uncomplicated bacterial pneumonia, although it can be helpful in more complicated cases. Thoracic ultrasound can be used to characterize peripheral areas of consolidation and to obtain fine-needle aspirates for cytology. Cytology is often helpful in distinguishing inflammation from neoplastic infiltration. In addition, sonographic evaluation is particularly

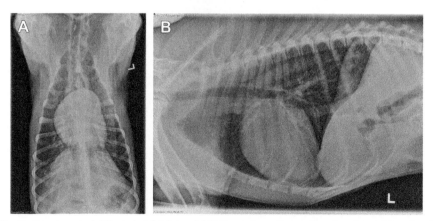

Fig. 2. Dorsoventral (*A*) and right lateral (*B*) thoracic radiographs of a dog with a focal, patchy, interstitial to alveolar pattern in the left cranial lung lobe. This dog was diagnosed with a foxtail foreign body, which was removed thoracoscopically via lung lobectomy.

Table 3
Differential diagnoses for specific radiographic patterns

Lobar Alveolar Consolidation	Focal Alveolar Consolidation
Aspiration pneumonia (cranioventral, right middle)	Airway foreign body
Lung lobe torsion (cranial)	Primary pulmonary neoplasia (caudal)
Atelectasis secondary to mucus plugging (right middle most commonly)	Metastatic neoplasia
	Noncardiogenic pulmonary edema

Diffuse Alveolar Pattern	Diffuse or Focal Interstitial Pattern
Acute respiratory distress syndrome	Early bacterial pneumonia
Congestive heart failure (perihilar in dogs)	Imminent congestive heart failure
Fluid overload	*Pneumocystis carinii* infection
Eosinophilic bronchopneumopathy	Inhalant toxicity (eg, paraquat)
Coagulopathy	Viral pneumonia
Metastatic neoplasia	

useful in the detection of superficial foxtail foreign bodies when they remain in the periphery of the lobe (**Fig. 3**).[10]

CT provides greater detail and resolution of lesions within the pulmonary parenchyma and gives the clinician better spatial information regarding the severity and extent of pulmonary involvement (**Fig. 4**). In some cases, CT can be useful to identify migration tracts associated with inhaled foreign bodies.[7] However, in most cases, general anesthesia is required for CT acquisition and prolonged recumbency can

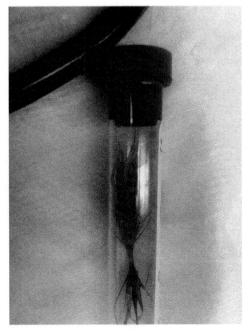

Fig. 3. A foxtail foreign body retrieved bronchoscopically from the left principal bronchus of a dog with chronic respiratory signs. Foxtails are endemic to the Western and Midwestern United States and are often associated with mixed aerobic, anaerobic, and fungal infections.

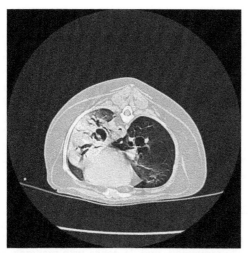

Fig. 4. CT image of a dog with severe, diffuse pneumonia resulting from a chronic foxtail foreign body (see **Fig. 3**). The foreign body was not visible on thoracic radiographs, but is clearly evident in the left principal bronchus on this image.

lead to atelectasis, which is difficult to differentiate radiographically from infiltrates. Repeating the CT in a different position after providing several maximal inspirations can alleviate atelectasis. Nuclear scintigraphy can be useful for the evaluation of ciliary dyskinesia, although secondary causes of mucociliary stasis (ie, infection with *Mycoplasma* or *Bordetella*, as well as exposure to smoke) must be excluded before assuming the diagnosis of PCD. Because of the time necessary for image acquisition, magnetic resonance imaging is not commonly used for the diagnosis of most respiratory diseases.

Bronchoscopic Evaluation

Examination of the trachea and bronchial tree should be performed systematically. The endoscopist should note the color and character of the mucosa and any airway sections, making sure to evaluate all branches of the lower airways for evidence of foreign bodies, bronchiectasis, or collapse (diffuse or focal changes). Airway mucosa in a normal animal should be pale pink with visible mucosal and pulmonary vessels. Airway bifurcations should appear as narrow, crisp mucosal margins.

Animals with pneumonia can have hyperemia of the epithelium, prominent mucosal vessels, and evidence of airway inflammation, appearing as rounded, thickened airway bifurcations and airway nodules. Airway secretions are usually opaque, viscous, and discolored (brown, yellow-green, or red tinged).

Airway Sampling

When available, BAL is preferred for collection of a lower airway sample rather than tracheal wash because the trachea and carina are not sterile, even in healthy dogs.[15] In addition, the sensitivity for detecting cytologic features of sepsis is greater with BAL than tracheal wash.[12] However, when only a tracheal wash specimen can be obtained, because of the lack of equipment for BAL or because of patient instability, collection of a lower airway sample is desirable to identify infecting bacteria and to determine appropriate antibiotic therapy through susceptibility testing.

BAL cell counts in animals with bacterial pneumonia are markedly higher than in patients with chronic bronchitis or other respiratory disease.[14] Septic, suppurative inflammation is a reliable indicator of bacterial pneumonia in dogs[14] and is likely to indicate bacterial pneumonia in cats. In those cases that lack evidence of airway sepsis (intracellular bacteria), BAL cytology generally reveals suppurative or mixed inflammation.[13]

In animals with suspected or confirmed foreign bodies, a BAL sample should always be obtained from the affected airway and submitted individually for cytologic analysis. Airway bacteria are more likely to be found in the cytologic sample from the site of the foreign body than from an alternate site.[8] Furthermore, cytology of BAL samples obtained from multiple lobes can reveal different findings, even in cases of sterile inflammatory diseases like feline bronchial disease, thus reliance on a single-segment BAL cytology could lessen the chance of yielding diagnostic results.[16]

Microbiology

Diagnosis of bacterial pneumonia relies on identification of septic inflammation in conjunction with a positive bacterial culture. Aerobic and *Mycoplasma* culture and sensitivity are typically requested, and, in cases with markedly purulent secretions or a history of known aspiration or foreign bodies, anaerobic cultures should also be requested. Samples should be refrigerated in sterile containers until submitted. If multiple alveolar segments are sampled during BAL, these are usually are pooled for culture submission.

Cultures should always be performed when possible in order to guide appropriate antimicrobial therapy. With the liberal use of antibiotics, increasing populations of resistant microbes are being identified, particularly in patients with hospital-acquired pneumonia.[17,18] However, airway samples cannot be collected in all animals and, in those instances, judicious use of antibiotics must be followed.

Common bacteria cultured from lung washes of cats or dogs with bacterial pneumonia include enteric organisms (*Escherichia coli*, *Klebsiella* spp), *Pasteurella* spp, coagulase-positive *Staphylococcus* spp, beta-hemolytic *Streptococcus* spp, *Mycoplasma* spp, and *B bronchiseptica* (**Table 4**).[4,13,27]

Pulmonary Function Testing

Arterial blood gas analysis is a useful test to measure the lung's ability to oxygenate. For patients with significant respiratory compromise, arterial blood samples ideally should be collected and analyzed to determine the severity of pulmonary disease.

Table 4	
Bacteria commonly isolated from airway samples of canine patients with pneumonia	
Organism	**Percentage of Isolates**
B bronchiseptica	22–49
E coli	11–17
Klebsiella pneumoniae	2–6
Pasteurella spp	3–21
Mycoplasma spp	30–70
Streptococcus spp	6–13
Staphylococcus spp	14
Anaerobes	5–17

Data from Refs.[4,13,26]

Furthermore, trends in arterial oxygen partial pressures can be used to track progression or resolution of disease. In many cases, blood gas analysis is not available or patient factors preclude the acquisition of samples. Pulse oximetry is a quick, noninvasive evaluation of oxygen delivery to body tissues that measures percentage of hemoglobin saturation with oxygen. It provides only a crude assessment of oxygenation and is subject to variability; however, trends in hemoglobin saturation can provide additional clinical support to progression or resolution of disease.

TREATMENT

Treatment of bacterial pneumonia varies considerably with the severity of disease, and appropriate antibiotic therapy is essential. The International Society for Companion Animal Disease is currently constructing guidelines for antibiotic therapy for respiratory infections. Pending those guidelines, antibiotic recommendations from previous literature should be considered (**Table 5**). For stable animals with mild disease, outpatient therapy consisting of administration of a single, oral antibiotic is often all that is necessary. Antimicrobial choices should ideally be based on culture and sensitivity results from airway lavage samples, although sometimes empiric therapy is more practical. Regardless, in cases of severe pneumonia, initial empiric therapy should be instituted while awaiting culture results. Antibiotics are typically administered for 3 to 6 weeks, and at least 1 to 2 weeks beyond the resolution of clinical and/or radiographs signs of disease.

Animals with more advanced disease require more intensive care, including hospitalization with intravenous fluids to maintain hydration. Adequate hydration is essential to facilitate clearance of respiratory exudates. Nebulization to create particles that enter the lower airways (<5 μm) can also enhance clearance of secretions. Nebulizer types include ultrasonic devices, compressed air nebulizers, and mesh nebulizers. Nebulization with sterile saline can be achieved by directing the hosing from the

Table 5	
Empiric antibiotic choice for patients with pneumonia	
Stable patient, mild clinical signs	Monotherapy: Trimethoprim sulfate 30 mg/kg PO every 12 h Amoxicillin–clavulanic acid 13.75 mg/kg PO every 12 h (dog) 62.5 mg PO every 12 h (cat)
Moderate clinical signs	Monotherapy: As listed earlier Dual therapy: Amoxicillin–clavulanic acid 13.75 mg/kg PO every 12 h (dog) 62.5 mg PO every 12 h (cat) And Enrofloxacin 10 mg/kg PO/IV every 24 h (dog) 5 mg/kg PO/IV every 24 h (cat) Or Amikacin 15 mg/kg SQ every 24 h
Critical patient, severe clinical signs	Dual therapy As listed earlier Monotherapy: Timentin-clavulanic acid 50 mg/kg IV every 6 h Meropenem 24 mg/kg IV every 24 h Imipenem 10 mg/kg IV every 8 h

Abbreviations: IV, intravenous; PO, by mouth; SQ, subcutaneous.

nebulizer into a cage or animal carrier covered in plastic. Depending on how viscous secretions are, therapy can be provided for 15 to 20 minutes 2 to 4 times daily. In many cases, nebulization coupled with coupage helps the animal expectorate airway secretions. Coupage is performed by cupping the hands and gently and rhythmically pounding on the lateral thoracic walls in dorsal to ventral and caudal to cranial directions. Coupage should not be performed in animals with regurgitation because any increase in intrathoracic pressure could exacerbate regurgitation and subsequent reaspiration.

Supplemental oxygen is necessary for animals with moderate to marked hypoxemia (documented by a Pao_2 less than 80 mm Hg or oxygen saturation via pulse oximetry less than 94% on room air) in conjunction with increased respiratory effort. Oxygen supplementation at 40% to 60% is provided until respiratory difficulty lessens and the animal can be weaned to room air. Animals with refractory pneumonia that fail to improve on supplemental oxygen can succumb to ventilatory fatigue and need to be referred to an intensive care facility for mechanical ventilation.

Administration of an oral mucolytic agent such as N-acetylcysteine can be useful for animals with moderate to severe bronchiectasis that are prone to recurrent pneumonia. Decreasing the viscosity of airway secretions might improve expectoration of fluid and debris that accumulates in dependent airways, although no published information is available on use of mucolytics in animals. N-acetylcysteine is typically not used via nebulization because of the risk of bronchoconstriction and epithelial toxicity. Under no circumstances are cough suppressants (such as butorphanol or hydrocodone) appropriate for use in the management of bacterial pneumonia, particularly when it is complicated by bronchiectasis. By decreasing the cough reflex, these drugs perpetuate retention of mucus, debris, and other material in the airways and therefore hinder clearance of infection. Also, furosemide should not be used because drying of secretions traps material in the lower airway and perpetuates infection.

In cases in which aspiration pneumonia is suspected, strategies should be used to reduce the chance of reaspirating through appropriate treatment of the underlying condition. With disorders of esophageal motility, upright feedings of either slurry or meatballs can enhance esophageal transit. Furthermore, diets low in fat can increase gastric emptying. In patients with refractory vomiting, antiemetic and prokinetic agents can be used to reduce the episodes of vomiting. Drugs like maropitant (Cerenia; 1 mg/kg subcutaneously once daily) or ondansetron (Zofran; 0.3–1 mg/kg intravenously or subcutaneously once to twice daily) act peripherally and centrally to decrease the urge to vomit and are safe to use in both cats and dogs.

The role of antacids in management of aspiration pneumonia remains controversial. By neutralizing the pH of gastric secretions, animals with refractory vomiting or regurgitation are less likely to succumb to chemical injury related to aspiration. However, in cases treated with acid suppression, the aspirant is likely to contain a greater concentration of bacteria that can colonize the lower airways and lead to bacterial pneumonia. No controlled studies have assessed the severity of aspiration pneumonia or the relative risk of using antacid therapy in dogs or cats.

Because radiographic findings lag behind clinical disease, recheck radiographs are not helpful early into the disease process, although they are useful to document resolution of disease and should be obtained within a week of discontinuation of antimicrobial therapy. In cases of refractory pneumonia, recheck radiographs midway through therapy can be used to assess resolution or progression of disease and help to guide further therapy.

In animals suspected of having contagious or multidrug-resistant pathogens, appropriate contact precautions should be used. Isolation gowns, examination gloves, and good hand washing technique along with appropriate quarantine facilities are essential to preventing transmission of disease to other patients or members of the health care team.

PROGNOSIS

Prognosis for animals with bacterial pneumonia varies depending on the severity of disease, the animal's immunocompetence, and the virulence of the infectious agent. In general, between 77% and 94% of patients diagnosed with pneumonia are discharged from the hospital.[4,19] No long-term studies assess the overall prognosis of patients with multidrug-resistant bacteria or recurrent pneumonia. The outcome associated with these cases presumably will be worse.

CASE STUDIES
Case Study 1

An 8-year-old female spayed Chihuahua mix presented for a wet cough.

History
Cough had been present for 4 months and there had been minimal response to antibiotics combined with a cough suppressant and no response to heart failure medication (furosemide, enalapril, and pimobendan).

Physical examination
Temperature (38.9°C [102°F]), pulse (140 beats per minute [bpm]), and respiratory rate (30 breaths per minute) were normal. No murmur was auscultated and lung sounds were normal.

Diagnostic evaluation
Chronic cough in a small-breed dog is often associated with airway collapse or chronic bronchitis; however, infectious and neoplastic disease must remain on the differential list. Congestive heart failure is unlikely given the lack of a heart murmur and the lack of response to diuretic therapy.

A white blood cell count was normal (5800 cells/μL) with 4400 neutrophils. Thoracic radiographs revealed scattered bronchial markings in the caudal thorax (**Fig. 5**). Fluoroscopic examination did not reveal evidence of tracheal or airway collapse. Laryngoscopy indicated lack of abduction of the arytenoid cartilages consistent with bilateral laryngeal paralysis. Secretions were evident throughout the upper and lower airways. Diffuse airway hyperemia and irregularities of the mucosa were apparent. BAL cytology was remarkable for septic suppurative inflammation, and bacterial cultures were positive for *Pasteurella*, *Mycoplasma* spp, and anaerobic bacteria, consistent with an aspiration cause.

Case Study 2

A 5-year-old male castrated domestic medium hair cat was presented for evaluation of acute respiratory distress.

History
Lethargy and anorexia had been noted 3 days before the onset of respiratory signs.

Physical examination
Temperature (38.7°C [101.6°F]) and pulse (210 bpm) were normal. Tachypnea was noted (respiratory rate, 60 breaths per minute) with increased respiratory effort on inspiration and expiration. Diffuse expiratory wheezes were auscultated.

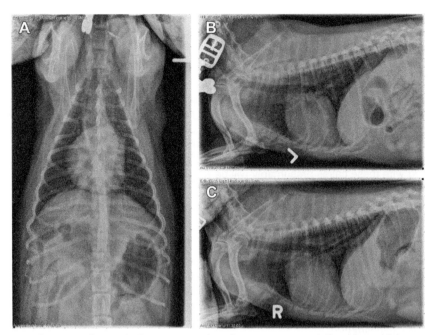

Fig. 5. Thoracic radiographs from case study 1 demonstrate a multifocal bronchial pattern throughout the caudal lung fields and a noticeable lack of alveolar infiltrates.

Diagnostic evaluation

Acute onset of respiratory difficulty in a cat is most commonly related to inflammatory airway disease. The physical examination is consistent with this diagnosis, although it is uncommon for affected cats to show lethargy and anorexia. Infectious and neoplastic diseases were also on the differential diagnosis list, along with aspiration and foreign body pneumonia.

Thoracic radiographs revealed a focal opacity in the left caudal lung lobe and a diffuse bronchial pattern (**Fig. 6**). Complete blood count revealed a normal white blood

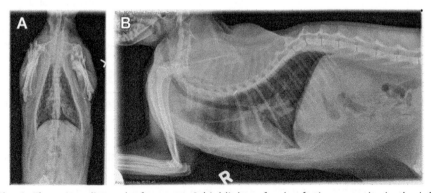

Fig. 6. Thoracic radiographs from case 2 highlight a focal soft tissue opacity in the left caudal lung fields along with a diffuse bronchial pattern and a scant pneumothorax. A left lateral radiograph was not obtained.

cell count (8500/μL) with a left shift (6800/μL neutrophils, 1000/μL bands). Bronchoscopy with lavage was performed. A moderate amount of airway hyperemia and edema was noted along with purulent material obstructing several airways. BAL cytology showed increased cellularity (1500, normal 500 cells/μL) with neutrophilic inflammation (84%, normal 5%–8%). Neutrophils contained dark blue granular debris, suspicious for sepsis. Aerobic and anaerobic cultures were negative but a pure culture of *Mycoplasma* was isolated on special medium. A diagnosis of mycoplasma bronchopneumonia was made.

REFERENCES

1. Leroy O, Vandenbussche C, Coffinier C, et al. Community-acquired aspiration pneumonia in intensive care units. Epidemiological and prognosis data. Am J Respir Crit Care Med 1997;156(6):1922–9.
2. Tart KM, Babski DM, Lee JA. Potential risks, prognostic indicators, and diagnostic and treatment modalities affecting survival in dogs with presumptive aspiration pneumonia: 125 cases (2005-2008). J Vet Emerg Crit Care (San Antonio) 2010;20(3):319–29.
3. Brownlie J, Mitchell J, Walker CA, et al. Mycoplasmas and novel viral pathogens in canine infectious respiratory disease. J Vet Intern Med (Seattle) 2013. Available at: http://www.vin.com/doc/?id=5820275.
4. Radhakrishnan A, Drobatz KJ, Culp WT, et al. Community-acquired infectious pneumonia in puppies: 65 cases (1993-2002). J Am Vet Med Assoc 2007; 230(10):1493–7.
5. Workman HC, Bailiff NL, Jang SS, et al. *Capnocytophaga cynodegmi* in a rottweiler dog with severe bronchitis and foreign-body pneumonia. J Clin Microbiol 2008;46(12):4099–103.
6. Tenwolde AC, Johnson LR, Hunt GB, et al. The role of bronchoscopy in foreign body removal in dogs and cats: 37 cases (2000-2008). J Vet Intern Med 2010; 24(5):1063–8.
7. Schultz RM, Zwingenberger A. Radiographic, computed tomographic, and ultrasonographic findings with migrating intrathoracic grass awns in dogs and cats. Vet Radiol Ultrasound 2008;49(3):249–55.
8. Epstein SE, Mellema MS, Hopper K. Airway microbial culture and susceptibility patterns in dogs and cats with respiratory disease of varying severity. J Vet Emerg Crit Care (San Antonio) 2010;20(6):587–94.
9. Craven DE, Hjalmarson KI. Ventilator-associated tracheobronchitis and pneumonia: thinking outside the box. Clin Infect Dis 2010;51(Suppl 1): S59–66.
10. Egberink H, Addie D, Belak S, et al. *Bordetella bronchiseptica* infection in cats. ABCD guidelines on prevention and management. J Feline Med Surg 2009; 11(7):610–4.
11. Kogan DA, Johnson LR, Jandrey KE, et al. Clinical, clinicopathologic, and radiographic findings in dogs with aspiration pneumonia: 88 cases (2004-2006). J Am Vet Med Assoc 2008;233(11):1742–7.
12. Hawkins EC, DeNicola DB, Plier ML. Cytological analysis of bronchoalveolar lavage fluid in the diagnosis of spontaneous respiratory tract disease in dogs: a retrospective study. J Vet Intern Med 1995;9(6):386–92.
13. Johnson LR, Queen EV, Vernau W, et al. Microbiologic and cytologic assessment of bronchoalveolar lavage fluid from dogs with lower respiratory tract infection: 105 cases (2001-2011). J Vet Intern Med 2013;27(2):259–67.

14. Peeters DE, McKiernan BC, Weisiger RM, et al. Quantitative bacterial cultures and cytological examination of bronchoalveolar lavage specimens in dogs. J Vet Intern Med 2000;14(5):534–41.
15. McKiernan BC, Smith AR, Kissil M. Bacterial isolates from the lower trachea of clinically healthy dogs. J Am Anim Hosp Assoc 1984;20:139–42.
16. Ybarra WL, Johnson LR, Drazenovich TL, et al. Interpretation of multisegment bronchoalveolar lavage in cats (1/2001-1/2011). J Vet Intern Med 2012;26(6): 1281–7.
17. Chalker VJ, Waller A, Webb K, et al. Genetic diversity of Streptococcus equi subsp. zooepidemicus and doxycycline resistance in kennelled dogs. J Clin Microbiol 2012;50(6):2134–6.
18. Foley JE, Rand C, Bannasch MJ, et al. Molecular epidemiology of feline bordetellosis in two animal shelters in California, USA. Prev Vet Med 2002;54(2):141–56.
19. Kogan DA, Johnson LR, Sturges BK, et al. Etiology and clinical outcome in dogs with aspiration pneumonia: 88 cases (2004-2006). J Am Vet Med Assoc 2008; 233(11):1748–55.
20. An DJ, Jeoung HY, Jeong W, et al. A serological survey of canine respiratory coronavirus and canine influenza virus in Korean dogs. J Vet Med Sci 2010;72(9): 1217–9.
21. McBrearty A, Ramsey I, Courcier E, et al. Clinical factors associated with death before discharge and overall survival time in dogs with generalized megaesophagus. J Am Vet Med Assoc 2011;238(12):1622–8.
22. Bedu AS, Labruyere JJ, Thibaud JL, et al. Age-related thoracic radiographic changes in golden and Labrador retriever muscular dystrophy. Vet Radiol Ultrasound 2012;53(5):492–500.
23. Watson PJ, Herrtage ME, Peacock MA, et al. Primary ciliary dyskinesia in Newfoundland dogs. Vet Rec 1999;144(26):718–25.
24. Watson PJ, Wotton P, Eastwood J, et al. Immunoglobulin deficiency in Cavalier King Charles spaniels with Pneumocystis pneumonia. J Vet Intern Med 2006; 20(3):523–7.
25. Jezyk PF, Felsburg PJ, Haskins ME, et al. X-linked severe combined immunodeficiency in the dog. Clin Immunol Immunopathol 1989;52(2):173–89.
26. Jameson PH, King LA, Lappin MR, et al. Comparison of clinical signs, diagnostic findings, organisms isolated, and clinical outcome in dogs with bacterial pneumonia: 93 cases (1986-1991). J Am Vet Med Assoc 1995;206(2):206–9.
27. Pesavento PA, Hurley KF, Bannasch MJ, et al. A clonal outbreak of acute fatal hemorrhagic pneumonia in intensively housed (shelter) dogs caused by Streptococcus equi subsp. zooepidemicus. Vet Pathol 2008;45(1):51–3.
28. Mellema M. Viral pneumonia. In: King LG, editor. Textbook of respiratory disease in dogs and cats. St Louis (MI): Saunders; 2004. p. 431–45.
29. Chalker VJ, Brooks HW, Brownlie J. The association of Streptococcus equi subsp zooepidemicus with canine infectious respiratory disease. Vet Microbiol 2003; 95(1–2):149–56.
30. Knesl O, Allan FJ, Shields S. The seroprevalence of canine respiratory coronavirus and canine influenza virus in dogs in New Zealand. N Z Vet J 2009;57(5):295–8.
31. Mitchell JA, Brooks HW, Szladovits B, et al. Tropism and pathological findings associated with canine respiratory coronavirus (CRCoV). Vet Microbiol 2013; 162(2–4):582–94.
32. Kawakami K, Ogawa H, Maeda K, et al. Nosocomial outbreak of serious canine infectious tracheobronchitis (kennel cough) caused by canine herpesvirus infection. J Clin Microbiol 2010;48(4):1176–81.

33. Keil DJ, Fenwick B. Canine respiratory bordetellosis: keeping up with an evolving pathogen. In: Carmichael LE, editor. Recent advances in canine infectious disease. International Veterinary Information Service; 2000.
34. Chalker VJ, Owen WM, Paterson C, et al. Mycoplasmas associated with canine infectious respiratory disease. Microbiology 2004;150(Pt 10):3491–7.
35. Priestnall S, Erles K. *Streptococcus zooepidemicus*: an emerging canine pathogen. Vet J 2011;188(2):142–8.
36. Foster SF, Martin P, Allan GS, et al. Lower respiratory tract infections in cats: 21 cases (1995-2000). J Feline Med Surg 2004;6(3):167–80.
37. Wood PR, Hill VL, Burks ML, et al. *Mycoplasma pneumoniae* in children with acute and refractory asthma. Ann Allergy Asthma Immunol 2013;110(5):328–34.

Exudative Pleural Diseases in Small Animals

Steven E. Epstein, DVM

KEYWORDS

- Pyothorax • Chylothorax • Bilothorax • Hemothorax

KEY POINTS

- Exudative pleural effusions have high total protein and high nucleated cell counts.
- Hemothorax is most frequently caused by trauma or a coagulopathy, with neoplasia, infectious causes, and lung-lobe torsion implicated less commonly.
- Pyothorax in dogs and cats can be successfully managed medically or surgically. Surgical indications include migrating foreign bodies or pulmonary abscessation.
- Chylothorax is a rare disease, and idiopathic effusion is the most common diagnosis. Surgical intervention is typically needed for resolution, and involves thoracic-duct ligation with pericardectomy or cisterna chyli ablation for optimal chances of success.

ANATOMY AND DEVELOPMENT OF PLEURAL EFFUSIONS

The pleural cavity, a potential space formed by the visceral and parietal pleura, is divided into a right and left pleural cavity separated by the mediastinum. There is controversy in dogs and cats as to whether the right and left pleural cavities communicate or are complete structures representing a barrier to movement of fluid from one side of the pleural cavity to the other.[1] Anatomists have described the mediastinum to be complete in the dog, although clinical experience suggests this might not be accurate. Infusion of saline unilaterally in dogs has resulted in bilateral distribution experimentally,[2] whereas infusion of air has been localized unilaterally in some experimental dogs.[3] Clinical experience would suggest that disease starting unilaterally can become bilateral or stay unilateral. This process likely indicates that some dogs and cats have a communication between the left and right pleural space, whereas in others it does not communicate, or that communications can be sealed because of disease.

In healthy animals a small volume of fluid is present in the pleural space to create minimal friction during movement of the lungs during respiration. The amount of fluid in normal dogs and cats is approximately 0.1 and 0.3 mL/kg body weight, respectively.[4] The amount of fluid present is related to Starling forces and removal of this fluid

Disclosures: None.
Department of Veterinary Surgical and Radiological Sciences, University of California–Davis, Davis, CA 95616, USA
E-mail address: seepstein@ucdavis.edu

Vet Clin Small Anim 44 (2014) 161–180
http://dx.doi.org/10.1016/j.cvsm.2013.08.005
0195-5616/14/$ – see front matter © 2014 Elsevier Inc. All rights reserved.

by pleural lymphatic drainage. Starling forces that promote development of pleural effusion include an increase in capillary hydrostatic pressure, a decrease in capillary colloid osmotic pressure, and an increase in permeability of the capillary wall (Box 1). Alterations in the first 2 features tend to lead to a transudate or modified transudate (Table 1).

Exudative effusions usually result from an inflammatory process within the pleural cavity that results in elaboration of cytokines or other vasoactive mediators. These substances lead to an increase in capillary permeability (filtration coefficient), allowing protein-rich fluid to enter the pleural space along with a variety of inflammatory cells. This initial inflammatory response can be derived from endogenous mediators (eg, chyle, neoplastic cells) or exogenous mediators (eg, bacteria, virus, or fungus). The lymphatic system is responsible for draining fluid formed within the pleural space. Obstruction, disruption, or decreased efficacy of the lymphatic drainage system can also result in exudative effusions.

CLASSIFICATION AND TYPES OF EFFUSIONS

Sampling of pleural effusion via diagnostic or therapeutic thoracocentesis is indicated to classify the fluid as pure transudate, modified transudate, or exudate, as outlined in Table 1. The main causes of exudative pleural effusions are listed in Box 2.

HEMOTHORAX
Diagnosis

There is no standardized definition of hemothorax in veterinary medicine, as the hematocrit in the effusion will depend on the peripheral circulating hematocrit. Hemothorax can be defined as a pleural-space effusion with a hematocrit that is at least 25% of the peripheral blood.[5] Iatrogenic hemorrhage caused by thoracocentesis can be differentiated from an existing hemorrhagic effusion by the presence of platelets and the lack of erythrophagocytosis.

Etiology

There is a multitude of causes of hemothorax in cats and dogs, the first of which to consider is blunt, sharp, or iatrogenic trauma. The history of the patient can be used to identify whether the patient was hit by a car, or had recent thoracic surgery, thoracocentesis, intrathoracic fine-needle aspirate, venipuncture, or jugular catheter placement. When there is no history of trauma, coagulopathies, neoplasia, lung-lobe torsion, or infectious causes can be considered.

Box 1
Modified Starling Law applied to the pleural cavity

Net filtration = LA $[(P_c - P_{pl}) - \sigma(\pi_c - \pi_{pl})]$

LA: filtration coefficient

P: hydrostatic pressure

c: capillary

pl: pleural liquid

σ: reflection coefficient to protein

π: osmotic pressure

Data from Lai-fook SJ. Pleural mechanics and fluid exchange. Physiol Rev 2004;84:385–410.

Table 1 Fluid type and characteristics			
Type of Effusion	Transudate	Modified Transudate	Exudate
Total protein (g/dL)	<2.5	2.5–7.5	>3.0
Total nucleated cell count (cells/μL)	<1500	1000–7000	>7000

Data from Rizzi TE, Cowell RL, Tyler RD, et al. Effusions: abdominal, thoracic and pericardial. In: Cowell RL, Tyler RD, Menkoth JH, et al, editors. Diagnostic cytology and hematology of the dog and cat. 3rd edition. St Louis (MO): Mosby; 2008. p. 235–55.

Disorders of either primary or secondary hemostasis can lead to hemothorax, with anticoagulant rodenticide intoxication being the most frequent coagulation disturbance encountered in clinical practice. In a study of noncoagulopathic spontaneous hemothorax in dogs, the most common cause was neoplasia (14 of 16 dogs).[6] Identified malignancies included hemangiosarcoma, mesothelioma, metastatic carcinoma, osteosarcoma, and pulmonary carcinoma.

Other causes of hemothorax are less common and include lung-lobe torsion, pancreatitis, and infectious or parasitic causes including *Streptococcus equi* subsp *zooepidemicus, Angiostrongylus vasorum,* spirocercosis, or *Dirofilaria immitis.*[7–9] Lung-lobe torsion as a cause of hemothorax has been reported in both dogs and cats.[10] Afghan Hounds and Pugs are overrepresented,[11,12] and the finding of hemothorax in these breeds warrants investigation of lung-lobe torsion as the underlying cause.

Treatment

Treatment of hemothorax is based on correcting the underlying cause if possible. For most traumatic cases, no specific treatment is indicated. If cardiovascular shock is present it should be treated immediately with fluid resuscitation. Respiratory distress should be alleviated with thoracocentesis. Only sufficient blood should be removed to maintain patient comfort because the remainder of red blood cells will be reabsorbed over time. If intrathoracic neoplasia is diagnosed in a location amenable to surgical removal, resection can be considered.

Secondary coagulopathies should be treated with fresh-frozen plasma to normalize hemostasis. As already indicated, limited thoracocentesis is recommended initially because blood will continue to effuse until the coagulopathy is corrected. Transfusion of red blood cells is sometimes needed to maintain an appropriate level of oxygen

Box 2 Exudative pleural effusions
Hemorrhage (dog and cat)
Bile (dog and cat)
Chyle (dog and cat)
Septic
Bacterial (pyothorax) (dog and cat)
Aseptic
Neoplasia (dog and cat, may also be modified transudate)
Feline infectious peritonitis (cat)

delivery. Specific treatment for an infectious disease is indicated when diagnosed. Animals with lung-lobe torsion require lung lobectomy to resolve clinical signs. Prognosis for hemothorax ranges from poor to excellent depending on the underlying cause.

BILOTHORAX

Bilothorax is a rare condition in both human and veterinary medicine, and has been reported in 4 dogs and 2 cats. In dogs, 2 cases were associated with gunshot injuries resulting in diaphragmatic tears, 1 case was due to traumatic bile-duct rupture despite an intact diaphragm, and the fourth was a postoperative cholecystectomy with intact diaphragm.[13–16] In cats, bilothorax was identified after thoracostomy-tube placement and subsequent pleurobiliary fistula in one cat, and after gunshot injury and a diaphragmatic tear in the other.[17,18]

Diagnosis of bilothorax is based on a ratio of bilirubin concentration in the pleural effusion to serum that is greater than 1:1. Development of bilothorax appears to occur through formation of a pleurobiliary fistula or in association with bile leakage into the abdomen. Bile can be carried across the intact diaphragm in the lymphatics, with subsequent damage and leakage into the pleural space.

Medical therapy includes placing a thoracostomy tube with frequent drainage to minimize the degree of pleuritis. Lavage of the pleural space with warm saline can be considered. If medical therapy fails or if a pleurobiliary fistula is identified, exploratory surgery is indicated. In veterinary medicine, bilothorax is apparently associated with an excellent prognosis, with all reported cases being successfully treated.

PYOTHORAX
Etiology: Dogs

Potential causes of pyothorax include migrating foreign material, penetration of bite wounds, hematogenous spread, esophageal perforation, parasitic migration, previous thoracocentesis or thoracic surgery, progression of discospondylitis, and neoplasia with abscess formation. The cause of pyothorax may or may not be identified. In dogs, identification of the cause has been reported in only 2% to 19% of cases.[19,20] When an underlying cause can be documented, the most common is a migrating grass awn or plant material. In a large-scale study of grass awn migration, approximately 3% of patients had intra-abdominal or intrathoracic migration.[21] The most common origin of pyothorax is likely to be regionally dependent (eg, grass awns or foxtails are common in California).

When a grass awn enters the mouth and migrates down the respiratory tree, it can carry oral microbiological organisms into the lower respiratory tract. The shape of the grass awn favors forward migration owing to barbing of the awn, and they often penetrate into the pleural space. The grass awn can then stay in the pleural space causing pyothorax, or migrate elsewhere (eg, retroperitoneal space or through the thoracic wall into the subcutis) (**Fig. 1**).[22]

Etiology: Cats

Reported causes of pyothorax in cats include parapneumonic spread, foreign-body migration, or penetrating thoracic wounds. The predominant cause of feline pyothorax is not clear at this time. There is common belief that the primary route of infection is through bite wounds from other cats. Support for this belief is based on data indicating that organisms isolated from feline pyothorax are similar to those found in bite-wound abscesses. Additionally, affected cats are 3.8 times more likely to live in a multicat than in a single-cat household,[23] and a seasonal association has been found, with

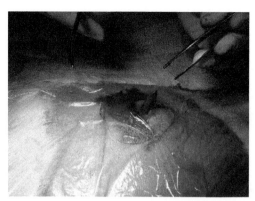

Fig. 1. Foxtail removed from subcutaneous swelling in a dog with pyothorax. (*Courtesy of* Dr Guillaume Hoareau, University of California, Davis, California.)

higher incidence in late summer or fall when enhanced outdoor activity would be expected. Recent history of wounds was also documented in up to 14.5% to 40% of cases in 2 studies.[23,24]

A more recent retrospective study suggested that 15 of 27 (56%) cats had parapneumonic spread of infection as the likely mechanism associated with pyothorax.[25] A case series describing pneumonectomy for parapneumonic spread in 4 cats was recently published that supported this etiology.[26] In 2 historical studies of pleural effusion, cats with pyothorax and an identified cause of effusion had pneumonia or a focal pulmonary abscess in 7 of 15 (47%) of cats.[27,28] At present the most likely cause of pyothorax has not been established, and there is evidence to support multiple causes in cats.

Diagnosis

Diagnosis of pyothorax is made based on cytologic examination of pleural fluid in combination with aerobic and anaerobic bacterial cultures. Gross characteristics of fluid that support the diagnosis of pyothorax include a turbid to opaque appearance in the presence of flocculent material. If anaerobic infection is present, there is often a malodorous smell. In a retrospective study of pleural and mediastinal effusions in dogs, pyothorax was the diagnosis in 13 of 81 animals (16%).[29]

Analysis of fluid typically reveals an exudate, and bacteria are often identified on microscopic evaluation (**Fig. 2**). In fact, bacteria were cytologically apparent in pleural fluid of 68% of dogs and 91% of cats in one study.[30] Mixed populations of bacteria are commonly seen. Identification of long filamentous bacteria is suggestive of involvement with *Actinomyces* or *Nocardia* species, which are often associated with grass awn migration and can be difficult to culture.[21] Bacteria may not be identified on cytology if antimicrobials have already been administered or if nonstaining infectious organisms (eg, *Mycoplasma*) are the causative agent. Nematode eggs have rarely been reported in pleural effusion of dogs.[31]

Microbiology

Multiple bacterial organisms have been cultured from dogs and cats with pyothorax. Aerobic, anaerobic, and mixed infections are documented most commonly.[19,30] *Pasteurella* spp are reported most commonly in cats, while in dogs, *Pasteurella* spp, enterics, anaerobes, and *Actinomyces/Nocardia* spp are the most common organisms

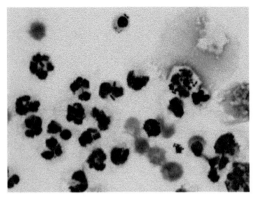

Fig. 2. Cytology of a dog with pyothorax showing both intracellular and extracellular bacteria. (Modified Wright Geimsa stain, 40× magnification.)

isolated. The population of bacteria present is likely regionally dependent in dogs, as grass awns (with associated *Actinomyces* infection) are overrepresented in some areas. **Box 3** lists other commonly identified bacteria.

Signalment

Cats and dogs with pyothorax tend to be younger, with an average age of 3 to 5 years, although it has been noted in a 1-month-old kitten.[32] Males of both species are overrepresented in multiple studies. Hunting dogs are overrepresented; however, no clear breed disposition in comparison with a general hospital population has been identified. No breed dispositions have been identified in cats, with domestic shorthairs and domestic longhairs representing the most frequent breed.

Box 3
Bacteria commonly associated with pyothorax in dogs and cats

Aerobes

    Pasteurella spp

    Escherichia coli

    Actinomyces spp

    Streptococcus canis

    Staphylococcus spp

    Corynebacterium spp (dog only)

Anaerobes

    Peptostreptococcus anaerobius

    Bacterioides spp

    Fusobacterium spp

    Porphyromonas spp

    Prevotella spp

Mycoplasma spp (cat only)

Data from Refs.[19,20,23,25,30]

Clinical Features

Animals with pyothorax have clinical signs related to pleural effusion and abscess formation. These signs can be either acute or chronic in duration. A restrictive breathing pattern can be noted in some animals, with tachypnea expected most commonly. Other common but nonspecific clinical signs include fever, anorexia, coughing, and lethargy. Fifty percent or less of cats with pyothorax will present with fever, showing that lack of an increase in body temperature should not exclude pyothorax from the differential list.[20,23,25]

Sepsis in cats is a common sequela to pyothorax, and in 29 cats with severe sepsis pyothorax was the most common underlying disease.[33] Moreover, in a separate retrospective study of cats diagnosed with pyothorax, more than 50% of cats had a concurrent clinical diagnosis of sepsis.[23] The proportion of dogs with sepsis caused by pyothorax is unknown at present.

Clinicopathologic Findings

Abnormalities in serum biochemical analysis are common in dogs and cats with pyothorax. Elevations in liver-enzyme activities, electrolyte disturbances, hypoproteinemia, and hypoglycemia or hyperglycemia are often documented. In a retrospective study, lower cholesterol concentration was a prognostic marker for survival in cats, although both groups had mean cholesterol concentrations within the reference interval, making this a dubious prognostic marker.[23] No biochemical abnormalities detected in dogs have been associated with survival.

Hematologic abnormalities of anemia and leukocytosis with neutrophilia are common in dogs and cats. In cats with pyothorax that died, lower leukocyte counts were observed compared with survivors, but this was nonsignificant when neutrophil counts were compared.[23] Dogs showed no association of survival with leukocyte count or band neutrophil count.[34]

Diagnostic Imaging

Thoracic ultrasonography is a frequently used technique to document moderate to large volumes of pleural effusion at the cage side, allowing the diagnosis of pleural effusion without moving a patient with respiratory compromise. With pyothorax, fluid is often echogenic, and fibrinous strands can be visualized between the pleural margins. Pulmonary foreign bodies can sometimes be detected,[22] and abscessation might also be visualized.

Thoracic radiographs are indicated to diagnose pleural effusion when ultrasonography is not available. However, if the respiratory distress is severe, therapeutic thoracocentesis should be considered before taking radiographs, or only a dorsal ventral projection should be obtained to confirm the diagnosis of pleural effusion without overly stressing the animals. It is important to remember, however, that in cases of small-volume effusion the ventrodorsal radiographic view has an increased ability to detect the fluid.

If imaging is performed before thoracocentesis, radiographs will demonstrate the classic signs of pleural effusion (retraction of lung borders from thoracic wall, interlobar fissure lines, loss of ventral cardiac silhouette, and so forth). Although most cases of pyothorax show bilateral effusion, unilateral effusion is not uncommon and is easily visualized on a dorsoventral radiograph (**Fig. 3**). If radiographs are taken before pleural drainage, they should be repeated after drainage to look for specific causes of pyothorax such as a mass lesion, focal pulmonary opacity, or foreign body.

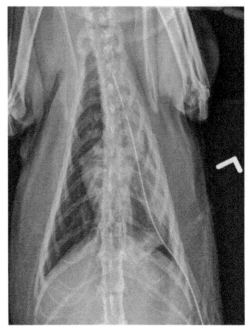

Fig. 3. Dorsoventral radiograph of a cat with unilateral pleural effusion secondary to pyothorax. A chest tube is appropriately placed in the left hemithorax to the level of the second rib.

Computed tomography (CT) is increasingly being used in veterinary medicine for the assessment of pyothorax. Recently a study of dogs and cats analyzing results of radiographs, CT, and ultrasonography in dogs and cats with migrating intrathoracic grass awns found a significant association between radiographic and CT localization and the gross site of lesions. Of note, CT was able to detect more sites of abnormalities and to trace the path of the foreign body more accurately than radiographs.[22] In a group of 8 dogs with pyothorax, CT localization of lesions was also highly correlated to surgical findings.[35] Therefore, CT can be useful in determining animals in which surgical therapy is indicated because of either a pulmonary abscess or a migrating foreign body (**Fig. 4**). At the author's institution (an area endemic for grass awns), CT is routinely used to screen for evidence of migrating grass awns in dogs with pyothorax.

Treatment

Treatment of pyothorax can be divided into medical or surgical management. Medical management involves thoracocentesis or placement of a thoracostomy tube. Surgical intervention usually refers to a median sternotomy and exploratory thoracotomy. The mainstays of treatment revolve around drainage of the purulent material, supportive care, and systemic antimicrobial therapy.

Depending on the likely cause of pyothorax and, thus, on geographic location, drainage alone by thoracocentesis or thoracostomy-tube placement can result in a good success rate in dogs (**Table 2**).[36] It should be noted, however, that studies with high success of medical therapy alone in dogs were performed in areas with low levels of migrating grass awns.[36] By contrast, Rooney and Monnet[34] found that treatment was 5.4 times as likely to fail in dogs treated medically as in dogs treated surgically, and 14 of 26 dogs (54%) had evidence of mediastinal or pulmonary lesions.

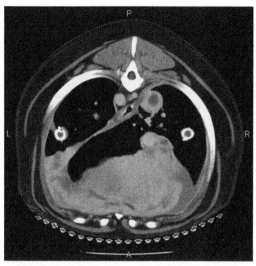

Fig. 4. Computed tomographic image of a dog with bilateral thoracostomy tubes and a pulmonary abscess secondary to a foxtail.

This result is in contrast to a more recent study by Boothe and colleagues,[19] whose findings failed to support the proposal of a better long-term outcome with surgical intervention. At present there is no consensus on the ideal therapy for all cases of canine pyothorax. Most clinicians would agree that if thoracic radiography or CT suggests pulmonary abscessation or migrating foreign material, surgical exploration of the thorax is warranted. However, successful treatment with thoracostomy-tube placement and supportive care could still be attempted when the owner is unable to pursue surgery.

Cats with pyothorax also have improved outcomes with either thoracostomy-tube placement or surgical exploration over thoracocentesis alone (**Table 3**). Although

Table 2		
Summary of outcome in canine pyothorax with various methods of treatment		
Authors,[Ref.] Year	**Procedure (n)**	**Survival to Discharge, n (%)**
Piek & Robben,[37] 2000	Thoracostomy tube (9)	9 (100)
	No evidence of migrating foreign body	
Demetriou et al,[20] 2002	Thoracostomy tube (29)	25 (86)
	Surgical exploration (7)	6 (86)
Rooney & Monnet,[34] 2002	Thoracostomy tube (7)	5 (71)
	Thoracostomy tube followed by surgery (12)	16 (84)
	Surgical exploration (7)	—
Johnson & Martin,[36] 2007	Thoracocentesis (16)	15 (94)
	No evidence pulmonary mass or consolidation	
Boothe et al,[19] 2010	Thoracocentesis (7)	2 (29)
	Thoracostomy tube (26)	20 (77)
	Surgical exploration (13)	12 (92)

Data from Refs.[19,20,34,36,37]

Table 3
Summary of outcome in feline pyothorax with various methods of treatment

Authors,[Ref.] Year	Procedure (n)	Survival to Discharge, n (%)
Demetriou et al,[20] 2002	Thoracostomy tube (11)	10 (91)
	Surgical exploration (3)	3 (100)
Waddell et al,[23] 2002	Thoracocentesis (39)	3 (8)
	Thoracostomy tube (48)	35 (73)
	Surgical exploration (5)	5 (100)
Barrs et al,[25] 2005[a]	Thoracocentesis (2) Small volume only	2 (100)
	Thoracostomy tube (19)	18 (95)
	Surgical exploration (1)	1 (100)
Crawford et al,[26] 2011	Surgery/Pneumonectomy (4)	4 (100)

[a] 5 cats died or were euthanized before initiation of therapy.
Data from Refs.[20,23,25,26]

there are reports of successful outcomes with single or repeated thoracocentesis, the largest retrospective study does not support this as a routine recommendation. Use of thoracostomy tubes for drainage is indicated in cats unless, similarly to dogs, pulmonary abscessation or migrating foreign material is suspected.

If thoracostomy tubes are chosen as the drainage technique of choice, the decision to place unilateral or bilateral tubes should be made on a case-by-case basis. The author typically will place one thoracostomy tube and drain the pleural space. Thoracic radiographs will be obtained and if effective drainage with one tube can be accomplished leaving minimal residual effusion, then only one tube is used. If a significant effusion is present in the hemithorax contralateral to the tube, a second thoracostomy tube can be placed. If the pyothorax is initially bilateral, the likelihood that bilateral thoracostomy tubes will be needed is greater, and some investigators recommend routine bilateral placement. Drainage from a thoracostomy tube can be accomplished by intermittent manual drainage or continuous suction, although the latter has not been shown to be advantageous.

There are 2 main methods of placement of a thoracostomy tube. A small-bore wire-guided chest drain can be placed via a modified Seldinger technique or a larger-gauge thoracostomy tube can be inserted in dogs or cats. One advantage to the small-bore (typically 14-gauge) thoracostomy tube is that it can be placed under sedation alone. Placement of this type of tube has been shown to be effective in a small group of dogs and cats with pyothorax.[38] However, obstruction of the tube by fibrin, and failure to completely drain the effusion are concerns with these small-bore catheters, and a larger-gauge trocar catheter (14–28F) is typically placed for animals with pyothorax, as described in **Box 4**.

Thoracic Lavage

Many investigators recommend thoracic lavage via a thoracostomy tube to facilitate evacuation of viscous pleural fluid. To date, no large-scale study in cats or dogs has evaluated outcomes with thoracostomy-tube placement comparing lavage versus no lavage, and no information is available on optimal thoracostomy-tube dwell time. In theory, the benefits of lavage include minimizing bacteria and inflammatory mediators in the pleural space, and increased removal of thick exudate that can plug the tube. Boothe and colleagues[19] showed improved outcome when pleural lavage was performed in preference to thoracocentesis only or thoracostomy tube without pleural

---

Box 4
Placement of trocarized thoracostomy tube by mini-thoracotomy

The animal is anesthetized and intubated to control ventilation and ensure adequate oxygenation. While in lateral recumbency, the thorax is clipped from the scapula to mid abdomen and the area is aseptically prepared. The skin over the lateral thorax is pulled cranially by an assistant and held in place. A thoracostomy tube is chosen that will easily fit through the intercostal space, and the length of the tube to be inserted is premeasured from the anticipated site of insertion to the second rib. It is imperative that all fenestrations in the tube be located within the thorax. The eighth or ninth intercostal space is located and a surgical drape is applied. A small skin incision, slightly larger than the diameter of the tube, is made at the junction of the dorsal one-third and ventral two-thirds margin of the lateral thorax. The subcutaneous tissue and muscle layers are bluntly dissected with a hemostat to the level of the pleura. The trocarized tube is then gently inserted into the thorax and the sharp tip of the trocar is retracted slightly back into the tube before advancement toward the elbow. The tube with partially retracted trocar is advanced the pre-measured distance directed towards the "up" elbow. After the tube is fully inserted, the trocar is removed and the thoracostomy tube is clamped to prevent entrance of air into the pleural space. The tube can then be connected to a closed adapter. Release of the cranially retracted skin creates a subcutaneous tunnel between the entry point in the thorax and the exit point in the skin. A purse-string suture is placed around the insertion site to assure a good seal, and the tube is secured in place with a finger-trap suture pattern.

---

lavage, but only 4 patients with thoracostomy tubes did not receive pleural lavage, making it difficult to extrapolate the results.

Addition of heparin to lavage fluid to assist with fibrin breakdown was evaluated in one canine study. Dogs with heparin (10 U/mL) added to their lavage fluid had improved short-term survival but no difference in long-term survival.[19] Because of only a short-term survival benefit, routine addition of heparin is not routinely recommended for pleural lavage. Addition of fibrinolytics, such as tissue plasminogen activator or urokinase, to lavage fluid is not routinely used in human medicine for thoracic empyema and cannot be recommended for veterinary patients.

If pleural lavage is chosen, warmed sterile isotonic saline is used at a dose of 10 to 20 mL/kg, infused slowly into the thoracostomy tube and left in the pleural space for 10 to 15 minutes before withdrawal. Typically less fluid is removed than is infused. Accurate record keeping of volume in and volume out should be performed to avoid fluid overload in the patient. Hypokalemia was documented in one cat undergoing pleural lavage.[25]

Indwelling thoracostomy tubes are generally removed when fluid production has decreased to 3 to 5 mL/kg/d and improvement is noted clinically, radiographically, and pathologically. Either ultrasonography or thoracic radiographs should be performed to confirm minimal effusion in the pleural space before withdrawal of the tube. Cytologic analysis of the fluid should demonstrate no evidence of infectious organisms, and neutrophils will be nondegenerate. In general, the neutrophil count will decline with successful treatment. However, this is not always a useful indicator of resolution of disease because when fluid production is minimal, there can be an artificial elevation of cellular concentration. The median duration of an indwelling thoracostomy tube has been reported as 5 to 8 days.[19,23]

Antimicrobial Therapy

Initial antimicrobial therapy is broad spectrum and is often administered intravenously. Given the variety of pathogens reported, final therapy should be based on culture and susceptibility results for the animal. However, initially, a β-lactam with β-lactamase inhibitor (amoxicillin/sulbactam) antimicrobial combination is chosen, because of its efficacy against *Actinomyces* spp as well as anaerobes. Therapy with enrofloxacin is often added for improved gram-negative coverage pending culture results.

Antimicrobial treatment is often long term, although there is little evidence to support this. It seems likely that animals treated medically would require longer therapy than those treated surgically, although this also has not been evaluated. One clinical approach is to have the patient return at 2-week intervals for clinical assessment and thoracic radiographs, and to treat with antimicrobials for an additional 2 weeks beyond resolution of radiographic signs. Mean duration of antimicrobial therapy in 2 studies on cats was 5 to 7 weeks.[20,25] The British Thoracic Society recommends treatment with oral antimicrobials for at least 3 weeks for humans with pleural empyema, with the ultimate duration based on clinical, biochemical, and radiologic response.[39]

Infusion of intrapleural antimicrobials has not been evaluated in veterinary pyothorax. However, it is not used in human medicine and is unlikely to be beneficial in veterinary patients. Systemic delivery results in adequate pleural concentrations for effective therapy.

Indications for Surgery

The main indications for exploratory thoracotomy are failure to respond to medical therapy, and diagnostic imaging findings supportive of mediastinal or pulmonary abscessation or migrating foreign material. Failure of medical therapy would include persistence of effusion despite thoracostomy drainage, persistence of infectious organisms despite appropriate antimicrobial therapy and thoracostomy drainage, or failure of clinical improvement in the first 72 hours. The presence of *Actinomyces* could be considered an indication for a thoracotomy owing to the association of migrating grass awns with this bacterium. It is important for clinicians to bear in mind that this bacterium can be difficult to isolate, and a presumptive diagnosis of *Actinomyces* is often made on cytology alone.

The goals at the time of surgery are to remove any inciting cause that can be discovered (eg, pulmonary abscess or foxtail), remove any necrotic material such as mediastinal or pulmonary tissue, and to break down any adhesions causing pocketing of fluid that cannot be drained by a thoracostomy tube.

Bronchoscopy

The role of bronchoscopy in pyothorax has not been well investigated in veterinary medicine. CT failed to detect all lesions in animals with pyothorax caused by migrating grass awns, and thus the primary purpose of bronchoscopy would be as an adjunct to CT for identification of foreign bodies.[22] As bronchoscopy has been shown to be successful in removal of foreign bodies in up to 76% of animals,[40] it should be considered before exploratory thoracotomy when a migrating grass awn is the suspected cause of pyothorax.

Prognosis

The prognosis for canine and feline pyothorax can be good with appropriate treatment. Ultimately it depends on the severity of clinical signs, and animals with severe sepsis have a worse prognosis than clinically healthy animals. **Tables 2** and **3** summarize survival data from the literature since 2000, and provide an overall survival of 83% in dogs and 62% in cats undergoing various treatment options.

CHYLOTHORAX

Chylothorax is an accumulation of chyle (lymph) within the pleural cavity resulting from impaired or obstructed lymphatic drainage. The primary lymphatic vessel within the thorax is the thoracic duct. The thoracic duct is the cranial continuation of the cisterna chyli, which returns lymph and chyle from the intestines, liver, and caudal half of the body. The thoracic duct typically converges with the venous system at the point where the internal and external jugular veins meet the cranial vena cava.

Etiology

Chylothorax can result from abnormalities of the lymphatic vessels, increased venous hydrostatic pressure at the level of the right heart, abnormal organ positioning, neoplasia, or idiopathic causes. Trauma to the thoracic duct is also reported to cause chylothorax; however, in experimental models of laceration and transection of the thoracic duct in dogs, sustained chylothorax was not observed.[41] Clinically, patients with thoracic-duct rupture are unlikely to develop significant pleural effusion and are not commonly seen. Other causes of thoracic-duct abnormalities include fungal granulomas, congenital abnormalities of the thoracic duct,[42] or transmural leakage across an intact but dilated vessel (lymphangiectasia).

Increased venous pressures can be due to cardiac disease, cranial vena cava obstruction, pericardial effusion, heartworm disease, or congenital cardiac abnormalities (tetralogy of Fallot, tricuspid dysplasia, double right ventricular outflow tract, or cor triatriatum dexter).[43–45] Abnormal organ positioning from peritoneal-pericardial diaphragmatic hernia or lung-lobe torsion has also been associated with chylothorax in the dog and cat.[11,46] However, the most common diagnosis in veterinary medicine appears to be idiopathic chylothorax.[47,48]

Diagnosis

Diagnosis of chylothorax is made on examination of pleural fluid. Typically it has a milky white appearance, and on cytologic analysis lymphocytes are the predominant cells, although with chronicity the number of nondegenerate neutrophils tends to increase. Small numbers of macrophages may also be noted. A Sudan stain can be used to verify lipid content in the sample. A definitive diagnosis is based on detection of a triglyceride level in fluid that is higher than serum on paired sample analysis.[49] If progressive disease and anorexia result in transudation of fewer lipids into the fluid, the effusion can lose its milky white appearance and appear more similar to serum. Therefore, in an anorectic patient with pleural effusion, chylothorax should remain on the differential list until triglycerides are measured or another disease is diagnosed.

Once chylothorax has been diagnosed, further diagnostic testing such as heartworm testing, echocardiography, thoracic ultrasonography, and radiography or CT should be performed to identify a potential cause. Abdominal imaging and assessment of gastrointestinal function can be used to investigate systemic lymphatic abnormalities. Owners should be questioned for any potential trauma in the history. If no identifiable cause is present, a diagnosis of idiopathic chylothorax is made.

Signalment

Chylothorax can occur in any breed of dog or cat, although the Afghan Hound is overrepresented among dog breeds because of the association of chylothorax with lung-lobe torsion.[11,50] In cats, Siamese are reported to be affected more commonly than other breeds.[51] Older cats develop chylothorax more often than younger ones, likely associated with the increased occurrence of cardiac disease and neoplasia in older cats.

Clinical Findings

Clinical signs of chylothorax are related to the development of pleural effusion. Animals can present with either acute or chronic disease. Abnormalities such as cardiac murmurs can be present depending on the underlying cause of the chylothorax. No consistent clinicopathologic abnormalities found on routine blood work are associated with chylothorax.

Medical Treatment

The cornerstone of medical management of chylothorax is control of the underlying condition; however, because most cases are idiopathic, specific therapy is rarely possible. Initial therapy involves removal of pleural effusion when respiratory distress is present. This action is unlikely to resolve the animal's condition, although there are rare reports of spontaneous resolution of chylothorax.[52] However, surgical options are generally not pursued immediately because of the chance for spontaneous resolution or the possibility that medical therapy will control the clinical signs.

Previously, medical management involved use of a reduced-fat diet supplemented with medium-chain triglycerides. However, in a study presented in abstract form, dogs fed a normal diet or a diet with reduced fat (20% and 2% of kcal) had no difference in the volume of lymph collected via thoracic-duct cannulation.[53] This finding has called into question the efficacy of a low-fat diet. Moreover, supplementation of medium-chain triglycerides is no longer recommended because these substances appear in thoracic duct lymph via absorption through the lacteals, and are not transported via the portal vein as originally thought.

Given the lack of specific medical management that is possible in most cases, alternative therapies can be used on a trial basis. Rutin is a nutraceutical purported to increase uptake of edema fluid by lymphatic vessels. Rutin has been evaluated in 3 reports, with 5 of 6 cats showing some degree of improvement.[54–56] The efficacy of rutin for idiopathic chylothorax in dogs has not been reported as yet. Octreotide is a somatostatin analogue that has been used in dogs and cats for the management of chylothorax. However, given its low success rate, expense, and parental route of delivery, it is not widely used.

Surgical Treatment

Thoracic-duct ligation is involved in the surgical treatment of idiopathic chylothorax; therefore, imaging of the duct is indicated before surgery. Preoperative imaging provides the surgeon with knowledge of the branching anatomy of the thoracic duct and allows ligation at an area of minimal branching, which is considered likely to optimize success of the surgery. The principle behind thoracic-duct imaging is injection of a contrast agent into a lymph node caudal to the thorax followed by radiographic or direct visualization of the thoracic duct.

The original description of mesenteric lymphangiography involved direct cannulation of a lymphatic vessel in the abdomen and injection of a contrast agent. Recently, minimally invasive or percutaneous techniques have been used. The ideal technique for visualization of the thoracic duct would seem to be CT. More branches of the thoracic duct can be identified by CT than with radiography when using popliteal lymphangiography.[57] Ultrasound-guided injection into the mesenteric lymph node and direct injection into the popliteal lymph node have been evaluated in dogs and cats.[57–61] Both techniques appear to be adequate for the visualization of the thoracic duct.[62] These techniques also can allow detection of thoracic lymphangiectasia if present (**Fig. 5**).

The choice of popliteal lymph node or mesenteric lymph node often depends on the skill level and comfort level of the operator. Mesenteric administration of contrast was successful in 8 of 10 dogs after 1 attempt while popliteal administration of contrast was successful in 8 of 11 dogs after 2 attempts; however, popliteal administration required less time than mesenteric administration and resulted in less discomfort.[63] At present, both sites seem able to produce diagnostic images.

Injection of methylene blue into the popliteal and mesenteric lymph nodes has also been attempted. The purpose of this is to colorize the thoracic duct to make it easier to identify at the time of surgery. Thoracic-duct coloration was identified with both techniques within 10 minutes of injection, and persisted for up to 60 minutes.[63]

Because of the inflammatory nature of chyle and the risks for the development of pleuritis and pericarditis, surgical intervention is recommended if chylothorax persists longer than 4 weeks despite medical therapy. Thoracic-duct ligation is the most common procedure used for the surgical treatment of idiopathic chylothorax in dogs and cats. The thoracic duct can be directly visualized and ligated along with each branch, or an en bloc ligation can be performed by clipping all of the structures in the caudal mediastinum dorsal to the aorta but ventral to the sympathetic ganglion.[64] This en bloc technique was evaluated in cadaveric dogs and was 93% successful in encircling all branches of the thoracic duct.[65] In clinical patients with chylothorax, ligation of the thoracic duct alone yielded a success rate of 50% to 59% in dogs and 14% to 53% in cats.

Because of its relatively low success rate, thoracic-duct ligation is usually combined with pericardectomy and/or cisterna chyli ablation. Studies from the last 10 years show similar success rates for surgical thoracic-duct ligation combined with pericardectomy and thoracic-duct ligation with cisterna chyli ablation. Thoracic-duct ligation combined with pericardectomy resolved the idiopathic chylothorax in 43 of 55 (78%) animals.[66–69] Thoracic-duct ligation combined with cisterna chyli ablation resolved idiopathic chylothorax in 23 of 27 (85%) patients.[69–71]

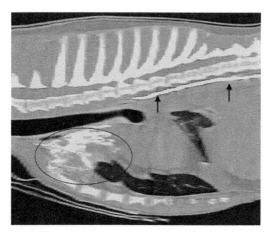

Fig. 5. Reconstructed computed tomographic image of a dog after ultrasound-guided mesenteric lymphangiography, demonstrating cranial mediastinal lymphangiectasia with leakage of contrast medium from the lymphatics into the cranial mediastinum (*oval*). Arrows highlight the thoracic duct.

Video-assisted thoracoscopic surgery (VATS) has also been used as a less invasive technique for thoracic-duct ligation and pericardectomy in dogs and cats.[72–74] With this procedure 13 of 15 (87%) patients had resolution of idiopathic chylothorax, making this a promising new technique. An alternative minimally invasive approach involving catheterizing the cisterna chyli and embolization the thoracic duct is being investigated at present.[75]

The addition of omentalization of the thorax to thoracic-duct ligation and pericardectomy has been investigated in 2 reports[76,77]; however, it does not appear to have an advantage over more traditional surgical approaches.

If surgical intervention does not resolve chylothorax, pleurodesis can be considered to create adhesions between the parietal and visceral pleura, although it has been challenging experimentally to achieve complete adhesions. An alternative to pleurodesis is placement of a pleural-peritoneal shunt to allow active or passive movement of chyle into the peritoneal space for resorption there. A PleuralPort (Norfolk Vet Products, Skokie, IL) can also be placed. This device is a thoracostomy tube attached to a titanium hub that is surgically placed into the subcutaneous space. Pleural effusion can then be aspirated directly by insertion of a needle into the hub.

SUMMARY

Successful management of an exudative pleural effusion requires an accurate diagnosis of the type of effusion present as well as identification of the underlying condition responsible for fluid accumulation. Prognosis can be favorable but expensive, and invasive techniques are often required for resolution.

REFERENCES

1. Evans HE. The respiratory system. In: Evans HE, editor. Miller's anatomy of the dog. Philadelphia: WB Saunders; 1993. p. 463–93.
2. Von Recum AF. The mediastinum and hemothorax, pyothorax and pneumothorax in the dog. J Am Vet Med Assoc 1977;171(6):531–3.
3. Moran JF, Jones RH, Wolfe WG. Regional pulmonary function during experimental unilateral pneumothorax in the awake state. J Thorac Cardiovasc Surg 1977;74(3):396–402.
4. Miserocchi G, Negrini D, Mortola JP. Comparative features of Staling-lymphatic interaction at the pleural level in mammals. J Appl Physiol 1984;54:1151–6.
5. Prittie J, Barton L. Hemothorax and sanguinous effusions. In: King LG, editor. Textbook of respiratory diseases in dogs and cats. St Louis (MO): Saunders; 2004. p. 610–6.
6. Nakamura RK, Rozanski EA, Rush JE. Noncoagulopathic spontaneous hemothorax in dogs. J Vet Emerg Crit Care (San Antonio) 2008;18(3):292–7.
7. Sasanelli M, Paradies P, Otranto D, et al. Haemothorax associated with angiostrongylus vasorum infection in a dog. J Small Anim Pract 2008;49(8):417–20.
8. Chikweto A, Bhaiyat MI, Tiwari KP, et al. Spirocercosis in owned and stray dogs in Grenada. Vet Parasitol 2012;190(3–4):613–6.
9. Byun JW, Yoon SS, Woo GH, et al. An outbreak of fatal hemorrhagic pneumonia caused by *Streptococcus equi* subsp. *zooepidemicus* in shelter dogs. J Vet Sci 2009;10(3):269–71.
10. Schultz RM, Peters J, Zwingenbuerger A. Radiography, computed tomography and virtual bronchoscopy in four dogs and two cats with lung lobe torsion. J Small Anim Pract 2009;50:360–3.

11. Neath PJ, Brockman DJ, King LG. Lung lobe torsion in dogs: 22 cases (1981-1999). J Am Vet Med Assoc 2000;217(7):1041–4.
12. Murphy KA, Brisson BA. Evaluation of lung lobe torsion in Pugs: 7 cases 1991-2004. J Am Vet Med Assoc 2006;228:86–90.
13. Guillaumin J, Chanoit G, Decosne-Junot C, et al. Bilothorax following cholecystectomy in a dog. J Small Anim Pract 2006;47:733–6.
14. Barnhart MD, Rasmussen LM. Pleural effusion as a complication of extrahepatic biliary tract rupture in a dog. J Am Anim Hosp Assoc 1996;32:409–12.
15. Bellenger CR, Trim C, Summer-Smith G. Bile pleuritis in a dog. J Small Anim Pract 1975;16:575–7.
16. Davis KM, Spaulding KA. Imaging diagnosis: biliopleural fistula in a dog. Vet Radiol Ultrasound 2004;45:70–2.
17. Wustefeld-Janssens BG, Loureiro JF, Dukes-McEwan J, et al. Bilothorax in a Siamese cat. J Feline Med Surg 2011;13:984–7.
18. Murgia D. A case of combined bilothorax and bile peritonitis secondary to gunshot wounds in a cat. J Feline Med Surg 2012;15(6):513–6.
19. Boothe HW, Howe LM, Boothe DM, et al. Evaluation of outcomes in dogs treated for pyothorax: 46 cases (1983-2001). J Am Vet Med Assoc 2010;236(6):657–63.
20. Demetriou JL, Foale RD, Ladlow J, et al. Canine and feline pyothorax: a retrospective study of 50 cases in the UK and Ireland. J Small Anim Pract 2002; 43:388–94.
21. Brennan KE, Ihrke PJ. Grass awn migration in dogs and cats: a retrospective study of 182 cases. J Am Vet Med Assoc 1983;182:1201–4.
22. Schultz RM, Zwingenberger A. Radiographic, computed tomographic, and ultrasonographic findings with migrating intrathoracic grass awns in dogs and cats. Vet Radiol Ultrasound 2008;49(3):249–55.
23. Waddell LS, Brady CA, Drobatz KJ. Risk factors, prognostic indicators, and outcome of pyothorax in cats: 80 cases (1986-1999). J Am Vet Med Assoc 2002;221(6):819–24.
24. Jonas LD. Feline pyothorax: a retrospective study of twenty cases. J Am Anim Hosp Assoc 1983;19:865–71.
25. Barrs VR, Allan GS, Martin P, et al. Feline pyothorax: a retrospective study of 27 cases in Australia. J Feline Med Surg 2005;7:211–22.
26. Crawford AH, Halfacree ZJ, Lee KC, et al. Clinical outcome following pneumonectomy for management of chronic pyothorax in four cats. J Feline Med Surg 2011;13:762–7.
27. Davies C, Forrester SD. Pleural effusion in cats: 82 cases (1987-1995). J Small Anim Pract 1996;37:217–24.
28. Hayward AH. Thoracic effusions in the cat. J Small Anim Pract 1968;9:75–82.
29. Mellanby RJ, Villiers E, Herrtage ME. Canine pleural and mediastinal effusions: a retrospective study of 81 cases. J Small Anim Pract 2002;43:447–51.
30. Walker AL, Jang SS, Hirsh DC. Bacteria associated with pyothorax of dogs and cats: 98 cases (1989-1998). J Am Vet Med Assoc 2000;216(3):359–63.
31. Klainbart S, Mazaki-Tovi M, Auerbach N, et al. Spirocercosis-associated pyothorax in dogs. Vet J 2007;173:209–14.
32. Gulbahar M, Gurturk K. Pyothorax associated with Mycoplasma sp and Arcanobacterium pyogenes in a kitten. Aust Vet J 2002;80(6):344–5.
33. Brady CA, Otto CM, Van Winkle TJ, et al. Severe sepsis in cats: 29 cases (1986-1998). J Am Vet Med Assoc 2000;217(4):531–5.
34. Rooney MB, Monnet E. Medical and surgical treatment of pyothorax in dogs: 26 cases (1991-2001). J Am Vet Med Assoc 2002;221(1):86–92.

35. Swinbourne F, Baines EA, Baines SJ, et al. Computed tomographic findings in canine pyothorax and correlation with findings at exploratory thoracotomy. J Small Anim Pract 2011;52:203–8.
36. Johnson MS, Martin MW. Successful medical treatment of 15 dogs with pyothorax. J Small Anim Pract 2007;48:912–6.
37. Piek CJ, Robben JH. Pyothorax in nine dogs. Vet Q 2000;22(2):107–11.
38. Valtolina C, Adamantos S. Evaluation of small-bore wire-guided chest drains for management of pleural space disease. J Small Anim Pract 2009;50:290–7.
39. Davies HE, Davies RJ, Davies CW. Management of pleural infection in adults: British Thoracic Society pleural disease guideline 2010. Thorax 2010;65(Suppl 2): ii41–53.
40. Tenwolde AC, Johnson LR, Hunt GB, et al. The role of bronchoscopy in foreign body removal in dogs and cats: 37 cases (2000-2008). J Vet Intern Med 2010; 24:1063–8.
41. Hodges CC, Fossum TW, Evering W. Evaluation of thoracic duct healing after experimental laceration and transection. Vet Surg 1993;22(6):431–5.
42. Schuller S, Le Garreres A, Remy I, et al. Idiopathic chylothorax and lymphedema in 2 whippet littermates. Can Vet J 2011;52:1243–5.
43. Fossum TW, Miller MW, Rogers KS, et al. Chylothorax associated with right-sided heart failure in five cats. J Am Vet Med Assoc 1994;204(1):84–9.
44. Dixon-Jimenez A, Margiocco ML. Infectious endocarditis and chylothorax in a cat. J Am Anim Hosp Assoc 2011;47(6):e121–6.
45. Singh A, Brisson BA. Chylothorax associated with thrombosis of the cranial vena cava. Can Vet J 2010;51:847–52.
46. Mclane MJ, Buote NJ. Lung lobe torsion associated with chylothorax in a cat. J Feline Med Surg 2011;13:135–8.
47. Ludwig LL, Simpson AM, Han E. Pleural and extrapleural diseases. In: Ettinger SJ, Feldman EC, editors. Textbook of veterinary internal medicine. St Louis (MO): WB Saunders; 2010. p. 1131–335.
48. Singh A, Brisson B, Nykamp S. Idiopathic chylothorax: pathophysiology, diagnosis and thoracic duct imaging. Compend Contin Educ Vet 2012;34(8):E2.
49. Fossum TW, Jacobs RM, Birchard SJ. Evaluation of cholesterol and triglyceride concentrations in differentiating chylous and nonchylois pleural effusions in dogs and cats. J Am Vet Med Assoc 1986;188(1):49–51.
50. Fossum TW, Brichard SJ, Jacobs RM. Chylothorax in 34 dogs. J Am Vet Med Assoc 1986;188(11):1315–8.
51. Fossum TW, Forrester SD, Swenson CL, et al. Chylothorax in cats: 37 cases (1969-1989). J Am Vet Med Assoc 1991;198(4):672–8.
52. Greenberg MJ, Weisse CW. Spontaneous resolution of iatrogenic chylothorax in a cat. J Am Vet Med Assoc 2005;226(10):1667–9.
53. Sikkema DA, McLoughlin MA, Birchard SJ, et al. Effect of dietary fat on thoracic duct lymph volume and composition in dogs. J Vet Intern Med 1993;7(2):119.
54. Gould L. The medical management of idiopathic chylothorax in a domestic long-haired cat. Can Vet J 2004;45(1):51–4.
55. Kopko SH. The use of rutin in a cat with idiopathic chylothorax. Can Vet J 2005; 46(8):729–31.
56. Thompson MS, Cohn LA, Jordan RC. Use of rutin for medical management of idiopathic chylothorax in four cats. J Am Vet Med Assoc 1999;215(3):345–8.
57. Singh A, Brisson BA, Nykamp S, et al. Comparison of computed tomographic and radiographic popliteal lymphangiography in normal dogs. Vet Surg 2011; 40:762–7.

58. Kim M, Lee H, Lee N, et al. Ultrasound-guided mesenteric lymph node iohexol injection for thoracic duct computed tomographic lymphography in cats. Vet Radiol Ultrasound 2011;52(3):302–5.
59. Johnson EG, Wisner ER, Kyles A, et al. Computed tomographic lymphography of the thoracic duct by mesenteric lymph node injection. Vet Surg 2009;38: 361–7.
60. Naganobu K, Ohigashi Y, Akiyoshi T, et al. Lymphography of the thoracic duct by percutaneous injection of iohexol into the popliteal lymph node of dogs: experimental study and clinical application. Vet Surg 2006;35:377–81.
61. Lee N, Won S, Choi M, et al. Thoracic duct lymphography in cats by popliteal lymph node iohexol injection. Vet Radiol Ultrasound 2012;53(2):174–80.
62. Millward IR, Kirberger RM, Thompson PN. Comparative popliteal and mesenteric computed tomography lymphangiography of the canine thoracic duct. Vet Radiol Ultrasound 2011;52(3):295–301.
63. Enwiller TM, Radlinsky MG, Mason DE, et al. Popliteal and mesenteric lymph node injection with methylene blue for coloration of the thoracic duct in dogs. Vet Surg 2003;32:359–64.
64. Singh A, Brisson B, Nykamp S. Idiopathic chylothorax in dogs and cats: nonsurgical and surgical management. Compend Contin Educ Vet 2012;34(8):E3.
65. MacDonald MH, Noble PJ, Burrow RD. Efficacy of en bloc ligation of the thoracic duct: descriptive study in 14 dogs. Vet Surg 2008;37:696–701.
66. Fossum TW, Merens MM, Miller MW, et al. Thoracic duct ligation and pericardectomy for treatment of idiopathic chylothorax. J Vet Intern Med 2004;18: 307–10.
67. Carobbi B, White RA, Romanelli G. Treatment of idiopathic chylothorax in 14 dogs by ligation of the thoracic duct and partial pericardectomy. Vet Rec 2008;163:743–5.
68. Adrega da Silva C, Monnet E. Long-term outcome of dogs treated surgically for idiopathic chylothorax: 11 cases (1995-2009). J Am Vet Med Assoc 2011; 239(1):107–13.
69. McAnulty JF. Prospective comparison of cisterna chyli ablation to pericardectomy for the treatment of spontaneously occurring idiopathic chylothorax in the dog. Vet Surg 2011;40:926–34.
70. Hayashi K, Sicard G, Gellash K, et al. Cisterna chyli ablation with thoracic duct ligation for chylothorax: results in eight dogs. Vet Surg 2005;34:519–24.
71. Staiger BA, Stanley BJ, McAnulty JF. Single paracostal approach to thoracic duct and cisternal chyli: experimental study and case series. Vet Surg 2011; 40:786–94.
72. Mayhew PD, Culp WT, Mayhew KN, et al. Minimally invasive treatment of idiopathic chylothorax in dogs by thoracoscopic thoracic duct ligation and subphrenic pericardectomy: 6 cases (2007-2010). J Am Vet Med Assoc 2012; 241(7):904–9.
73. Allman DA, Radlinsky MG, Ralph AG, et al. Thoracoscopic thoracic duct ligation and thoracoscopic pericardectomy for treatment of chylothorax in dogs. Vet Surg 2010;39:21–7.
74. Haimel G, Liehmann L, Dupre G. Thoracoscopic en bloc thoracic duct sealing and partial pericardiectomy for the treatment of chylothorax in two cats. J Feline Med Surg 2012;14(12):928–31.
75. Singh A, Brisson BA, O'Sullivan ML, et al. Feasibility of percutaneous catheterization and embolization of the thoracic duct in dogs. Am J Vet Res 2011;72(11): 1527–34.

76. Stewart K, Padgett S. Chylothorax treated via thoracic duct ligation and omentalization. J Am Anim Hosp Assoc 2010;46:312–7.
77. Bussadori R, Provera A, Martano M, et al. Pleural omentalization with en bloc ligation of the thoracic duct and pericardiectomy for idiopathic chylothorax in nine dogs and four cats. Vet J 2011;188:234–6.

Index

Note: Page numbers of article titles are in **boldface** type.

A

Aelurostrongylosis
    feline asthma *vs.*, 93
Airway collapse, **117–127**. *See also* Tracheal (airway) collapse
Airway sampling
    in bacterial pneumonia evaluation, 151–152
    in CCB, 111–112
Allergy testing
    in feline asthma evaluation, 96
Alveolar to arterial oxygen gradient
    in pulmonary gas exchange evaluation, 9–11
Anatomic dead space, 14
Antibacterial(s)
    in feline chronic rhinitis management, 41
Antibiotic(s)
    in pyothorax management, 171–172
    in tracheal (airway) collapse management, 125
Antihistamine(s)
    in feline chronic rhinitis management, 45
Antiinflammatory agents
    in feline chronic rhinitis management, 45–46
Antitussive agents
    in tracheal (airway) collapse management, 124–125
Antiviral agents
    in feline chronic rhinitis management, 43–44
Arterial blood gas analysis
    in IPF evaluation in WHWTs, 133–134
    in pulmonary gas exchange evaluation, 7–9
Aspergillosis
    feline, **51–73**
        causes of, 52–53
        classification schemes, 52
        clinical presentation of, 58
        diagnosis of, 60–66
            biochemistry in, 60
            biopsy procedures in, 63–65
            hematology in, 60
            histopathology in, 65–66
            imaging in, 62–63
            serology in, 61–62
        differential diagnosis of, 58–59
        epidemiology of, 53–56

Vet Clin Small Anim 44 (2014) 181–190
http://dx.doi.org/10.1016/S0195-5616(13)00218-0
0195-5616/14/$ – see front matter © 2014 Elsevier Inc. All rights reserved.

vetsmall.theclinics.com

Printed and bound by CPI Group (UK) Ltd, Croydon, CR0 4YY

12/10/2024

01773480-0003